# The Second Season

# The Second Season

## LIFE, LOVE, AND SEX— WOMEN IN THE MIDDLE YEARS

*Estelle Fuchs*, Ph.D.

ANCHOR PRESS / DOUBLEDAY
GARDEN CITY, NEW YORK
1977

The Anchor Press edition is the first publication
of THE SECOND SEASON.
Anchor Press edition: 1977

Library of Congress Cataloging in Publication Data

Fuchs, Estelle.
Second season: life, love, and sex—women in the middle
years.

Includes bibliographical references and index.
1. Middle age. 2. Middle age—Sexual behavior.
3. Women—Sexual behavior. 4. Menopause. I. Title.
HQ1221.F78      301.41'2
ISBN: 0-385-09760-3
Library of Congress Catalog Number 77-70897

mw 4/78  3908

TO
MY MOTHER

# Preface

This is a book designed to present a rational, enlightened view of the physiological and cross-cultural components of women's experience with middle age and the universal fact of menopause. While of primary interest to women, it should as well be interesting to men concerning a period of women's lives shrouded in myth, ignorance, misunderstanding, and apprehension; fleshing out gaps in training and understanding common among physicians, psychiatrists, employers, husbands, lovers, sons, etc. Most important, it should be an invaluable source of reliable information for women.

My own personal interest in the subject stems from the time I first matured. Abundantly available was literature on menstruation, anatomy, contraception, pregnancy. But menopause was invariably dismissed in a sentence, or at most a very brief paragraph, with the implication that "pause" ended everything discussed in the voluminous pages preceding. There were in the overheard conversations of "older" women the intimations of "hot flashes," a reference here and there to hysterical or depressed women, and, more recently, in the hormone vendors' advertisements in the medical periodicals, unnecessarily gruesome implications of withering away. Yet nowhere has there been readily available material where these negative notions could be tested, material that was clear, informative, and based on reliable data.

But there is more to this period of life than physiology. In literature and the mass media middle-age menopausal women have been treated, more often than not, as annoying and irrelevant. As my career as an anthropologist developed, it became increasingly clear that the highly variable social roles (romantic attractiveness, economic and political power, etc.) played by mature women in various cultures and in different periods of time contrasted sharply with the constricted view of female middle age prevalent in this society.

My experience both as a woman and as a professional anthropologist and educator led me to the conviction that a volume which brought together a cultural and physiological examination of middle-aged women was necessary.

I owe a debt of gratitude to Loretta Barrett, my friend and editor at Doubleday-Anchor, for her persistent encouragement which convinced me to undertake the effort this book entailed. To my husband, Willy, I wish to express profound thanks for the many ways in which he made it possible for me to attend to the task. The skill of Rita Roth in preparing the manuscript is deeply appreciated. Thanks also to Lela and my friends at Elia for their *joie de vivre*, an inspiration at all times.

ESTELLE FUCHS
*Mykonos, Greece*
1977

# Contents

# Contents

# The Second Season

# I

# Middle Age—Where It's At

Humans belong to a curious species—always seeking to explore, discover, learn. The antics of the chimps in the zoo as they respond to their environment amuse us; we take for granted the probing curiosity of our infants and ourselves as we go through life.

Inquisitive as we are about so many things, most of all we seem to be interested in people, searching for answers about mankind's relationship to the universe and to others. And in our time, perhaps more than ever before in history, we enjoy the luxury of exploring what is probably the most interesting subject of all—our individual selves.

Who am I? What am I? Where have I been and where am I going—*in my own life?* are the questions we ask ourselves almost from the earliest moments of our consciousness as we move beyond childhood. At adolescence these questions take on great significance as we test ourselves in the many possible relationships we have with people about us—playing the many changing roles, searching for a pattern of identity. And always who we are does not come simply from ourselves. We are of course our bodies, but our *personhood* is inextricably bound up with how others treat us and our vision of their perception; and with where we fit in the social group, the position we are in, and how we are supposed to behave in that position.

Our lives move so swiftly through time. In disbelief, women find themselves approaching forty and the premenopausal decade. Menopause and the decade following also seem to roll swiftly by. These are precious years—as are all the years on earth. Women in our time, in the modern world, search to live those middle years fully, to experience the wonders and joys of living, to not settle for inevitability and a life they cannot control, a life which they may or may not find pleasing, but at least one about which they themselves have made some decisions.

It is not surprising then, that as mid-life approaches women seem more eager than ever to reassess their lives, to make decisions about themselves and their futures. Tradition used to make these decisions for most of us—tradition still does for many—but women in today's world have extraordinary choices opening up, choices for which experience from the past does not seem an adequate guide. How can a woman know who she is and what she might do in a world that seems to turn things topsy-turvy overnight? What is being a middle-aged woman, *now* and for the *future*, all about?

What is it to be middle-aged? You'd think it would be easy to say. But what are we talking about? The body? The mind? The social creature?

Even the body confuses our efforts to be simple. It is sobering to think that the auditory ossicles of our ears are adult size before we are born; our brains often stay alert long after our limbs begin to creak. Women are told they can expect to live past seventy-five; that places middle age at thirty-seven, far too young even for the census takers to acknowledge that as a mid-point of our lives. Women begin to have the capacity to reproduce around the age of thirteen; it ends around fifty. Does that make fifty old? Or is thirty-seven again the middle age of our lives? The census takers use the figures of forty-five to fifty-four and fifty-five to sixty-four for mid-life; the Social Science Research Council and its team of prestigious social scientists speak of the years forty to sixty as marking mid-life.[1]

And age is so relative. To a nineteen-year-old girl, a man of twenty-five is old; to a forty-five-year-old woman, a man of forty is "young." In a society that values the wisdom of old people, a person of forty is still immature; in one that values youth, forty is "over the hill."

And sex—what is middle-aged for a woman is sometimes earlier than for a man when so often she is more valued for youth than he. But men die sooner. Are they really middle-aged earlier—while women last longer both in years and sexual vigor?

Cultures define middle age differently. So much depends on the roles that are played—are we middle-aged when new grandparents, do we stay young so long as we are not? Some languages have a word for middle age and one for old age—among some people you are old as soon as you are widowed, regardless of age.

Does menopause mark middle age? In some societies it is the station stop of old age, among others there is no concern—there isn't even a word for it—and femininity and activity go on and on.

Is middle age an attitude? Does willingness to learn to be flexible, to partake with vigor and joy of the choices open to us in life keep us from being old? We all know children who seem old and older people who seem so young. We may be too old for playing jacks, but young for golf and dancing and swimming. There are generational differences—some generations turning away from the world as they age, others partaking actively of it. Is middle age a time when reassessments are made and values re-examined and new roles assumed—does this happen once, many times over, or never in our lives? Is middle age the time we recognize that life is limited and time precious?

No one definition applies to all women or to all men everywhere. In our time and our experience, however, middle age is an ever-growing, significant period in the lives of women. Women are no longer precipitously plunged from their adulthood into old age, just as children in the modern world are no longer plunged from childhood into adulthood—we allow them a long period of adolescence and youth. Today, middle age is an ever-enlarging period, extending through at least two decades and probably longer.

Are there more or less of us at middle age? Over 21 per cent of Americans are between the ages of forty-five and sixty-four years—forty-two million people—more than half of whom are women! An ever-increasing number of people will be swelling the ranks of the middle-aged as the post World War II babies move inexorably through their thirties and into their forties and beyond.

To the woman of sixty, the forty-year-old is young, but the forty-year-old, nonetheless, is conscious of entering her mid-life and the premenopausal decade. A woman past fifty is hardly old and is increasingly conscious of that fact as she experiences the post-menopausal decade. And women in their early sixties, given health and pleasure in living, know that they are really not old, nor do they see themselves in the same category as those fortunate women who live into their seventies and eighties. There is plenty of time to be old. And so, for the modern woman, mid-life can encompass as much as a quarter of a century, plenty of time in which to grow, experience, and partake of the sometimes sad, sometimes joyous experience of living.

# Women and Sex—Here to Stay

In the pop culture of the Western world, the ideal image of feminine sexual attractiveness is usually that of the young, lithe, white, and more often than not blond beauty. Our popular novels have women in their twenties punctuating their other mundane activities by frequent popping in and out of bed with their lovers. Few of the glamorous movie stars who have won Academy Awards played women of middle age. An award for such a characterization was given Beatrice Straight in 1977 for her role in the popular film *Network*. But even here, the woman portrayed was the older wife abandoned by her husband for a much younger woman.

Although men experience some of the same bias against older persons as do women, there is no comparison in the way they are regarded in the popular culture. Despite the notion of "dirty old man" applied to older men interested in sex, middle-aged men are expected to—are indeed encouraged to—continue flirtations with the girls. There is no particular prejudice against men marrying women much younger, and therefore supposedly more sexually active than older women who are "tired," although the admiration and applause given men able to acquire young women is sometimes punctuated with the warning "she'll kill him." For Frank Sinatra to marry a Mia Farrow, younger than his daughter, hardly raises an eyebrow.

For a man to play a "fathering" role to a wife or mistress is compatible with what men are supposed to be in this culture: protective, supportive, stable, and economically responsible figures. "Mothering" a husband or lover, on the other hand is viewed as ludicrous and improper, for the traditional female role is one of nurturer of children, not of adult males.

But the cat has finally been let out of the bag. There is now ample evidence that female sexuality does not decline precipitously with middle age—on the contrary, apparently rising in intensity after the age of thirty-five well into the forties. The evidence comes to us from both biological and cultural sources, and it demonstrates that older women can not only be active and interested in their sexuality—even more so than younger women and men their age—but they also can be sexually attractive and stimulating to men.

For one thing, women, by the very nature of their anatomy, are capable of more sexual activity than men throughout their lives. Perhaps no one could describe this fact more vividly than America's great humorist Mark Twain, who wrote in the very irreverent, posthumously published *Letters from the Earth:*

> During twenty-three days in every month (in the absence of pregnancy) from the time a woman is seven years old till she dies of old age, she is ready for action, and *competent*. As competent as the candlestick is to receive the candle. Competent every day, competent every night. Also, she *wants* that candle—yearns for it, longs for it, hankers after it, . . .
>
> But man is only briefly competent; and only then in the moderate measure applicable to the word in *his* sex's case. He is competent from the age of sixteen or seventeen thenceforward for thirty-five years. After fifty [sic] his performance is of poor quality, the intervals between are wide, and its satisfactions of no great value to either party; whereas his great-grandmother is as good as new. There is nothing the matter with her plant. Her candlestick is as firm as ever, whereas his candle is increasingly softened and weakened by the weather of age, as the years go by, until at last it can no longer stand, and is mournfully laid to rest in the hope of a blessed resurrection which is never to come.
>
> By the woman's make, her plant has to be out of service three days in the month and during a part of her pregnancy.[1]

About men, he wrote that they set the rules for women ". . . without consulting the woman, although she has a thousand times more at stake in the matter than he has."

> His procreative competency is limited to an average of a hundred exercises per year for fifty years, hers is good for three thousand a year for that whole time—and as many years longer as she may live. Thus his life interest in the matter is five thousand refreshments, while hers is a hundred and fifty thousand; yet instead of fairly and honorably leaving the making of the law [of monogamy] to the person who has an overwhelming interest at stake in it, this immeasurable hog, who has nothing at stake in it worth considering, makes it himself!
>
> You have heretofore found out, by my teachings, that man is a fool; you are now aware that woman is a damned fool.[2]

It has taken the pioneering studies by Kinsey and Masters and Johnson to proclaim to the world what Mark Twain kept hidden from publication till after his death: Healthy women are capable of intercourse till their last breath, including sexual excitement, and resolution through orgasm. Masters and Johnson tell us that "there is no time limit drawn by the advancing years to female sexuality." They speak of ". . . significant sexual capacity and effective sexual performance among women 40 to 78."[3] Their significant work belies the mythology that for physical or physiological reasons, coital satisfaction decreases considerably after the normal menopause. Where a marked decrease in satisfaction occurs, it is usually the result of emotional factors, or the result of the self-fulfilling prophecy that it will occur.

But what of her sexual attractiveness to men? Aren't young women more stimulating and desirable to men than their older sisters?

It is very difficult to measure sexual attractiveness in biological terms. What is attractive or stimulating to a man is so often the result of what he has learned to believe is a desirable female. The tremendous value placed on the young, the firm, and the fair in American culture, for example, is so strong as to make it appear "natural" that men be attracted physically to such women. But compare this emphasis with that of other societies, or even among some men in our own who resist the current fad, who prefer the dark and voluptuous; to whom young, firm, and fair are simply skinny, pale, and juvenile.

The slender, sinewy models in ads for cosmetics, perfume, etc., who project an image of sensuality for us are the very antithesis of "sex appeal" elsewhere. Among the traditional Ibo of Nigeria, for example, in the past, girls at puberty were isolated away from the group before being presented publicly as available for marriage. During this period of isolation they did no work and were well fed—fattened for their debut. The plumper they were, the more desirable did the girls appear to their potential mates. And many a plump European or American has discovered that her sexual stock goes up in a country like Mexico. Papago Indians in the American Southwest tend to favor well-rounded women, but their neighbors, the Apache, lean toward the slender. One usually thinks of Asians as slim, but the admired Buddha is always portrayed with ample proportions.

But while it doesn't take too much of a stretch of the imagination to understand that Siberians might prefer cuddling with someone with enough flesh to really hold onto during their cold winter nights, the matter of age and sex is something different.

This view of the undesirability of older women is so pervasive in Western society that it is difficult for Western observers to see younger men with older women without inferring some ulterior motives on the part of the male. Usually, the snickers imply that the man is either a gigolo, being paid for his attentions, or that somehow he has snagged a wealthy widow or divorcee for the comforts her money will provide for him.

Even that early cautious observer of nature, the great botanist and naturalist Linnaeus, when twenty-five years of age, could not resist implying such motives while visiting among the Lapps of Lapland, in northern Sweden. Back in 1732 he wrote:

> I sat with my legs crossed, to the right of the entrance. Opposite me was an old woman with one leg straight, the other bent. She wore a silver belt, and her dress came no lower than her knees; her grey hair was hanging down; her face was wrinkled and her eyes bleary; her features were typically Lapp, and her fingers big and heavy . . . Besides her sat her husband, a young man of about thirty-eight who had married this old hag ten years since for the sake of her reindeer.[4]

Yet, here again, the evidence from other cultures—and indeed from the behavior of some within our own—indicates there is nothing "natural" about the young female being preferred above the older.

Despite the fact that it is extremely difficult for Europeans to comprehend, the conceptions of sexual attraction can be reversed as regards age. Among the traditional Lovedu, a Bantu people of Southern Africa, for example, marriages usually were arranged between persons of similar age. As has usually been the case in all societies, these marriages were for the establishment of relations between two sets of families as well as for the purpose of procreation. The Lovedu accepted the fact that sexual adventure and compatibilities may be sought outside of marriage, and so it was the married, rather than the unmarried, who had their lovers. Significantly, it was the *older* women who frequently had their liaisons with the young married men, and these men sought their adventures with women who might well be their mothers or grandmothers.[5]

Among the Coast Salish of the Pacific Northwest, it also was not unusual for young men to engage in romantic courtships with post-menopausal women.[6]

And why shouldn't an older woman be attractive to men, including men younger than herself? She, if healthy and physically active, is more likely to have both social and sexual skill, to have fewer inhibitions and problems to work through than younger women. In addition, it is useful to remember, she is less likely to involve a young man in unexpected pregnancies and other such complications. As an experienced woman she can skillfully induct young men into the art of love-making. To a man closer her age, she shares the experience of a generation and is potentially able better to relate to his perceptions and concerns.

In the United States some 5 per cent of the men aged forty-five to sixty-four are married to women in the age bracket ten years above theirs, while the overwhelming majority marry women slightly younger than themselves.

It is clear, however, that there is enormous prejudice within our culture against accepting older women as sexually as desirable as younger women. The prejudice has ancient roots. Freud spoke of the Oedipus complex to describe a pathological attachment of the son to the mother. Yet, in ancient Greece, it was the young Oedipus who, returning to Thebes, was attracted to and married Jocasta, old enough to be his mother, but whom *he did not know* was his mother. He suffered the punishment of the Greek gods for this unforgivable act. And Phaedra, too, fell in love with Hippolytus, son of the man she was to marry. The gods punished the unlucky young man as well, and poor Phaedra hanged herself in remorse. But rarely are older men so punished for their liaisons with women young enough to be their daughters.

The reasons for this cultural prejudice are complex, but a primary cause is probably the importance of marriage to women capable of childbearing. Marriage without procreation has usually not been acceptable, even for aging males, throughout history. Barrenness is frequently a calamity and an acceptable reason for divorce. Romantic involvements with older women simply upset the applecart in regard to the perpetuation of the society. And just to make sure, plenty of support on the side of younger women has been given in the form of religious sanctions and popular opinion.

But the ability to bear children and the ability to enjoy and engage in sex are two different things. Where childbearing is not considered important—as it frequently is to people in modern society who have had as many or few children as they wanted, when they wanted them—sex takes on more the function of play, "fun and games," if you will, than ever before. Human evolution has extended the period of play for mankind, both in the prolonged state of childhood, and the continuation of sexuality past the point of desired or possible reproductive functions.

Some human societies permit a great deal of sex play among children before reproductive age, and there does seem to be some evidence that the women of these groups, with the added sexual experience and fun in their childhood, experience more clear-cut orgasms during their adult years. Women of cultures with more restrictive attitudes seem to experience more difficulty with their sexuality.

Victorian traditions were extremely restrictive toward sex—sex as play was clearly forbidden the young, and sex in marriage was viewed as having only the function of inducing pregnancy. One shudders to think that some readers took literally the advice offered in the sex manual of the 1800s, the very opposite of the advice in today's manuals which go to the questionable extreme of prescribing ecstasy as necessary and, with proper techniques, always possible.

For example, the Victorian sex manuals of the nineteenth century advised women in general to contain their emotions and sensuality. They advised that the practice of reading the romantic novels of the era were the prime cause of uterine diseases. They warned women that the stimulation to their emotions and passions would cause uterine congestion, displacement, weak backs, painful menstruation, and most of the complications of menopause![7]

Some of these manuals warned that males had an aggressive nature, and that it was essential for females to remain cold, passive, and indifferent—to have no sex desire. One 1850 manual even warned that "voluptuous spasms" would cause a weakening and relaxing of the female which tended to cause her to be barren. In a peculiar twist of logic, the manual urged that in order to insure that the primary function of marriage be realized, i.e., pregnancy and childbearing, that the couple maintain separate bedrooms![8] (One is reminded with some sadness of the small bedroom used by Eleanor Roosevelt flanked on one side by that of her mother-in-law, and on the other by Franklin, at the Roosevelt Hyde Park Estate, and one wonders how much of their married life together was affected by the persistence of Victorian sex morality as it applied to the proper lady.)

On the whole, the ideal morality extolled by these sex manuals was that sex in marriage existed solely for the purpose of procreation, that sensuality and joy in sex represented a loss of dignity for the woman. It is impossible, of course, to know actually how many nine-teenth-century women followed the prescriptions of these self-appointed advisors on sexuality, or how many women, in giving vent to their sexual natures, were burdened with guilt and fear of the consequences of their behavior.

How different from Victorian morality is the attitude of the peoples of the Caucasus Mountains in Soviet Georgia who believe: "Sex . . . is guiltless and unrepressed. It is neither projected nor sublimated into work, art, or religious-mystical passion. It is not an evil to be driven from one's thoughts, but a pleasure to be regulated for the sake of health, and it improves with age—like a good wine."[9]

While we've come a long way since the restrictive attitudes promulgated by Victorian morality, nevertheless there still is in the culture an attitude that somehow male sexuality is more urgent and more persistent than that of the females. And there is still a lag in the incorporation of current knowledge in the texts used to teach young gynecologists and other doctors. It seems, however, that the women are changing their perceptions of their innate sexuality, thanks either to changes in society or information from the mass media. While at one time *Lady Chatterley's Lover* and *Ulysses* were collector's items, known to the few *cognoscenti*, anyone can pick up a copy of *Fear of Flying* almost anywhere, including the corner drug store, and read an account of open, accepted, feminine sexual adventure. And current sex manuals stress "joy" for both female and male.

These changed attitudes have had their effect on women of menopausal age as well as the young. Magazines such as *Vogue* and *Harper's Bazaar* tell in a chic way that women in their forties are "better than ever" and run special issues to proclaim the news. And, it appears women are more and more aware that what Kinsey has said—"there is little evidence of any aging in the sexual capacities of the female until late in her life"—has implications for their life style.

Drs. Leon and Shirley Sussman, Director and Associate Director of the Human Sexuality Center of the Long Island Jewish-Hillside

Medical Center in New York, report that they do not see women
feeling so badly about age and sex anymore. On the contrary, they
see women of menopausal age lively, active, and even eager. Perhaps
this generation of women missed out in their twenties and thirties—
many were separated from men during the Second World War,
many made early impetuous marriages, many did not work out their
sexual inhibitions until their forties. Now they seem ready to make
up for the past. What seems unfortunate to these researchers is that
many men are not as ready as the women are for a reinvigorated sex
life—perhaps because of early traumas in the marriage which are
difficult to overcome, perhaps because of their own problems with
sexuality in middle age.

Kinsey tells us that the female develops sexual urges more slowly
than does the male. He places the peak of male sexual prowess at age
seventeen, whereas girls do not begin to mature sexually until the
late teens or early twenties. Girls continue to increase their sexuality
slowly and steadily, and while the male's sexual powers are waning,
hers are maintaining their steady level well into her fifties and sixties.

How much of the slower development of female sexuality is due to
the cultural prejudice in the direction of inhibitions, which are overcome with experience as women reach their thirties and forties, is
difficult to say. Far from being "over the hill" or "tired" the woman
approaching and going through her menopause is likely to experience
a great resurgence in sexual interest and practice. She is, like the proverbial "vintage wine," happily improving in her sexual skill and
pleasure with age. It is at these ages, with children grown and out of
the house, there is often a resurgence of sexual interest and activity
between husband and wife—the second-honeymoon phenomenon.
For others, this is a period of sexual experimentation and fulfillment
outside of a marriage that might bear too many scars to overcome.
Some even suggest that such experimentation renews sexual interest
in their marriage.

Researchers at Duke University in North Carolina have also found
that women's rates of interest and activity as regards sex do not fall
off with increasing age. Yet, they found that fewer women than men
were sexually active after the age of sixty.[10] This probably reflects
both cultural attitudes against sexuality for women at advanced ages,
as well as the fact that women in middle age and after have fewer
male partners available to them due to the higher death rate among

men. There are twenty-two million women aged forty-five to sixty-four in this country, for example, compared with twenty million males. This means ninety-seven men for every one hundred women. The men are more likely to be married and some to women below the age of forty-five, and some (hardly all) unavailable for extra-marital sex. This puts older women at a distinct disadvantage—sexually—although considering the alternative, the higher death rate of men, they can't really complain.

Most significantly, the researchers at Duke University found that for the vast majority of older persons, sex continued to play an important part in their lives. By age fifty, about one half of their sample reported some decline in their sexual activity, but others reported an increase. And by age seventy, when most reported some decline, there still was a minority reporting an increase! It appears that the availability of an interested sexual partner is the major factor enabling persons to continue regular sexual relations into old age.

Mark Twain's welcome glorification of the female anatomy and its potential for everlasting sexual readiness, of course has to be tempered by reality. Despite her anatomical availability, a woman's sex life is affected not only by the availability of partners, but also her physical health. And no woman can go fornicating throughout her days and nights uninterruptedly without concern for infection and possible injury to sensitive tissues.

Age is a factor in these considerations, although none of them, given current medical knowledge, need interfere with her biological potential for sexuality into old age, and especially not at middle age. Dr. William Masters and Ms. Virginia Johnson, writing in *Human Sexual Response* point out that the sexually active woman "suffering from all of the vaginal stigmas of sex-steroid starvation still will retain a far higher capacity for sexual performance than her female counterpart who does not have similar coital opportunities." There is no reason, they emphasized, "why the milestone of the menopause should be expected to blunt the human female's sexual capacity, performance, or drive."[11]

Among the Nzakara, a people living on the Ubangi River in Eastern Africa, there is agreement with the Masters and Johnson attitude that practice keeps one young sexually. The Nzakara have no room for single women. They believe that a woman who no longer has a husband immediately becomes old!

For some women, for example, the degree of lubrication of the vagina is somewhat decreased. Lubricating creams or jellies or, if necessary, locally applied estrogen creams (which do not carry the same dangers of internally administered hormones) easily correct this situation. The vagina may become less elastic, but this hardly interferes with her enjoyment of sex—and since the elasticity functions to facilitate stretching of the vagina in childbirth, there is really little need at this age for a very elastic vagina. Some women and men are concerned that a less elastic vagina interferes with the sexual pleasures of the partners, especially when the vagina is large and the man's penis small. But Masters and Johnson have shown us that the contrary can be the case, for imaginative and skillful love-making can position the partners in such a way as not only to correct the disparity in size, but to add zest to love-making. Any change in the size of the clitoris—it may become smaller in some women—does not seem to be significant. They also tell us in their invaluable study, *Human Sexual Inadequacy*, that regular usage—continued and regular intercourse—helps keep the vagina youthful and that women who continue active sexual lives have vaginas that do not constrict significantly in size, continue to lubricate well, and that orgasms continue to be good.[12]

Certain physical conditions, such as prolapse of the uterus, can interfere with a continuing sex life. But these usually can be corrected and these are not conditions confined to older women—they can occur at any age, especially after childbirth.

Mark Twain's admonition to women that they are damned fools still seems worthy of attention. It appears that the attitudes toward female sexuality are changing only slowly. For example, a recent examination of twenty-seven gynecology textbooks written between 1943 and 1972 indicate that they continue to be written from a traditional male viewpoint.[13] They, on the whole, do not include the findings of Kinsey and Masters and Johnson to any considerable degree. In their study, Diana Scully and Pauline Bart found that half the texts repeated old falsehoods such as that the male sex drive is stronger than the females'; that women are interested in sex for procreation, not for recreation (obviously, if women want sex only to mother offspring, this eliminates the woman at menopause and beyond as a sexual person); and that most women are frigid and do not enjoy intercourse. It hardly seems likely, in the future, that such cavalier attitudes toward female sexuality can continue in the medical literature used to teach our doctors now that the biological, scientific evidence on sexuality is becoming better known to the lay public.

In his enormously popular book, *Everything You Wanted to Know About Sex but Were Afraid to Ask,* David Reuben, M.D. (a psychiatrist, not a gynecologist) did a disservice to women in his description of what would happen to them as a result of menopause. After first saying that sex at middle age was great, he then proceeded to describe a list of horrors that were to befall women.[14] Curiously enough, the description seemed almost a verbatim recital of the propaganda advertisements of the estrogen-producing drug companies who were engaged in the campaign to foist regular estrogen replacement therapy on all women during the 1960s and '70s. The symptoms he described do occur—but in the rare medical disorder known as *adrenogenital syndrome.* They are not typical of the healthy woman.

The biological evidence is accumulating to justify the conclusion that menopause, in the healthy woman with opportunity for continuing sexual activity, does not mean an end to female sexuality. On the contrary, her biological and anatomical superiority to the male in regard to intercourse is much in her favor during the middle years and beyond.

It is difficult to imagine that the postwar generation, with its freer sexuality and improved information will approach menopause with the willingness to forego continued sexuality.

Still, for many women, both in our culture and in others around the world, the end of childbearing has been directly associated with the end of femininity and frequently the end of sexuality. Rural women in Jamaica speak of the loss of their "health of flowers" and their "turning from the world" toward community and religious service. Moslem women can often anticipate divorce and replacement by younger wives, with no further opportunity of intercourse. And the Tiwi women of Melville Island, north of Australia, know that their opportunity for sexual intercourse decreases markedly at the end of their childbearing period, reversing the causation by believing that it is this end of intercourse which induces menopause rather than vice-versa!

In our own society the cultural attitudes that favor the young as desirable, as well as the biological reality of fewer males to females at increasing ages, also decreases the opportunity for continued sexuality. In as curious a twist of logic as that used by the Tiwi, our culture teaches us that menopause causes the end of the woman's sexual nature rather than the facts that cultural attitudes and male mortality combine to make opportunities for sex decline. The evidence seems to be that fewer and fewer women are accepting this attitude about themselves, refusing to define themselves as asexual after childbearing ceases.

It might be asked then, why is it that everywhere it seems to be the case that men are dominant and women subordinate, with men defining women's sexual role for them? In almost every human society the work that men and women do is judged this way, with men's work viewed as more important, and this is so even when men's work in one culture is the work that women do in another. And if, in reality, women are even more "competent" sexual creatures than men, as Mark Twain discerned and as Kinsey and Masters and Johnson have documented, why is male sexuality so often viewed as the more aggressive, the more vigorous?

Structural anthropologist Lévi-Strauss, who so heavily influenced the work of the renowned feminist Simone de Beauvoir, has offered a somewhat controversial theory to explain this.[15] He says that in the universal human experience there is a difference between what is nature and what is cultural, or imposed by man, and that culture dominates nature. In this order of things, women are viewed as closer to nature, the "raw," as opposed to men who are closer to culture, "the cooked." Lévi-Strauss supports this dichotomy by pointing to women's body functions as more obviously "nature"—they menstruate, they bear and suckle young. Man, on the other hand, transcends nature through "existence," goal-oriented activities which make him rise above the restrictions of the natural world. Lévi-Strauss condescends, however, to grant that woman after all is also a person with a consciousness—but she remains an intermediate between culture and nature. In a curiously ethnocentric recounting of what Western culture has defined woman to be, he sees that woman's social role, therefore, is to be in the realm of domesticity, nursing, cooking. He speaks of woman's psyche as lending itself to greater emotionality and irrational thinking. Yet he does not explain why it is in the Middle East that women are considered to be the more practical, pragmatic, and thus worldly, as compared with their men, who are allowed greater expression of emotionality and religious ardor. And there are some people, such as the Siriono of Brazil, who regard nature, the "raw," as maleness, as opposed to culture, the "cooked," as femaleness.[16]

In the Western world, too, there is a degree of contradictory evidence to Lévi-Strauss' theory. Women represented the cultural influence in European courtly love. And throughout Western culture there is the notion, as expressed in the Victorian sex manuals, that males have an aggressive animal, sexual nature and it is necessary and natural for women to remain cold, passive, and indifferent. When Captain Bligh and his men of the English ship *Bounty* landed on Tahiti back in 1789 they found people to whom such a definition of female sexuality was incredible. So incredible, indeed, that the men of the *Bounty* found it impossible to give up this surfeit of sexual riches offered by willing Tahitian women and return to England.

There seems to be a strange contradiction in the titillation men receive from their fantasy of the insatiable, ever-competent sexual female, as described by Mark Twain, and emphasized by Lévi-Strauss in his theory that man everywhere perceives women as nature, and the view that men are the sexual aggressors as opposed to female frigidity and temperance. Yet there may be no contradiction at all. It could be that this very fear of the insatiable and perpetually receptive female has, for their own protection, caused men to surround women with innumerable taboos and restrictions in regard to their sex lives.

But, as usual, contradictory views of woman prevail—she is either sexually voracious and irresponsible and must be restrained, or she is defined as frigid and sexually unresponsive to eager males. Traditional Moslem society regarded women as sexually irresponsible. Thus, the women were secluded in a harem, or women's quarter of the house, and were required to wear veils, following the injunction of the Koran that commanded the women not to display adornments to any but their husbands and nearest relatives. It certainly seems simpler for men to define women as sexually wanting, while the limitations are really more true of the male, but painful to accept.

Indeed, as Mark Twain so irreverently suggested, monogamy is more restrictive on women, sexually, than on men, given the biological potential. Of course, the matter is hardly that simple. Actually, there are very few societies in the world that permit women to marry several husbands (although often women are permitted to have more than one lover besides her husband). The practice of marrying several men is known as polyandry. A classic example of such a custom is to be found among the Toda peoples of India, a poor dairy herding group. There a woman married a group of brothers, who cared for the herds, in a practice called fraternal polyandry. Her primary task was to care for the house and to bear children. The brothers solved the issue of their marital rights rather simply; while one brother visited the wife, he left his spear outside the hut as a signal to his brothers to insure no interruption of connubial privacy. As far as what happened to the extra women is concerned, until the interference of modern government and Western religion, the Toda simply killed unwanted baby girls.

More often than not, however, where plural marriage does exist it usually is in the form of polygyny; that is, the man marries several wives. Everyone is familiar with the glamorous harem of the Middle East or the image of the sexy concubine in old China. But usually where men marry more than one woman, these wives are useful not only as sex partners and childbearers but also in the economic production of the household, and where it occurs, it is usually the richer men who have access to more than one wife. It is not unusual for the first wife to approve the acquisition of others—it gives her company, extra help, and greater social status. In some places in West Africa, for example, she even raises money for the bride-price for co-wives.

It takes elaborate etiquette and maneuvering for a man to behave in such a way that his various wives don't feel neglected and cause him aggravation. I recall a conversation held with a young man and his half sister from a Moslem family in Somalia. Both argued that their mutual father loved their respective mothers the most of all of his four wives. Each asked the other to present the evidence. It turned out that father, when visiting each of these two wives, pretended to be ill so he could stay several extra nights. He had cleverly employed a tactic to keep these two wives blissfully thinking each was the favorite. It probably was the case that he did the same with the remaining two. In any event, his sensibilities for the feelings of his wives did not put him above divorcing the eldest wife—mother of the young man—in order to make room in his permitted Moslem allotment of four for a woman younger than the boy's half sister, to insure the continued growth of his progeny.

By far the larger number of peoples in the world practice monogamy, with one man marrying one woman. In the Western world, where monogamy is reinforced by legal restrictions and religious sanction, men of means have always been known to acquire mistresses, and serial monogamy—that is, one wife at a time aided by the institution of divorce—legalizes access to more than one mate during a lifetime. What is curious, however, is that there generally has been a tendency to recognize male philandering as fairly common, but with the usual "blinkers on" it was sort of assumed that the women available to such men were the divorced or widowed, or the single younger girls not yet married. There is now plenty of evidence that not only married men are off to their affairs, but so are their wives, including wives well into their forties and fifties.

Male fantasy about the voracious female, based on reality or not, may be one cause for men establishing domination and defining women as sexually inferior to themselves. But it does seem more logical to believe that marriage customs and preference for younger women in marriage, as well, are based on the real need of societies to produce offspring to perpetuate themselves. During much of man's four- to six-million-year history as an evolving species, and during the past thirty-five thousand years or so of the life of our own anatomically modern species on earth, this was by no means a simple matter. Death in childbirth was not uncommon, infant mortality was high, but more important, the cultural skill to acquire adequate food and protection to support more than the smallest of bands took millennia to acquire. Life expectancy was limited, and the numbers who survived beyond menopause relatively small. It is only in our era that hundreds of millions of women can look forward to one third of their lives beyond menopause. And with that much time left, it is illogical to connect sex only with childbearing.

It seems far more sensible for the play aspects of sex now to take on greater significance. A woman's physiology, given reasonably good health, need not interfere. None of the things that *might* happen to some women—a little more time to be aroused, maybe fewer multiple orgasms, perhaps a smaller clitoris, or a vagina which requires some lubrication, greater attention to the possibility of infection—are enough to counteract the continuing potential for pleasure in her sexuality. The absence of a male partner, a real possibility, is one major threat, since many women find no enjoyment in masturbation or in lesbian relationships. Another major threat is a cultural attitude, accepted by some men *and* by some women as well, unfortunately, that perpetuates the notion of the close of sexuality at menopause.

Modern women more and more are casting off this stereotypical view of themselves as sexless, as they search for ways to enjoy sexual companionship in their mid-lives.

# Men and the Middle Years

I was forty years old and my husband forty-six when the eccentric behavior began. An otherwise reasonable and family-loving man suffered,
not depression as we understood it, but rage, fatigue, incommu-
nicability, suspicion, hostility. But every incident was my fault supposedly; I was the woman and I was alleged to be in the change of
life. . . . Unfortunately doctors, psychiatrists, men in general, have
kept it all under the rug where they have swept it themselves. They are
in terror of the truth of acknowledging a condition which affects their
behavior beyond their control, but which they readily ascribe to
women without mercy. . . . (Is there a male menopause or climacteric?) What does it matter what you call it, if it's there?

Anonymous letter, New York *Times*,
February 25, 1973

Do men have a menopause? Do they experience a mid-life crisis com-
bining hormonal and cultural changes that lead them to experience a
mid-life crisis, complete with a menopausal syndrome? What is the
male climacteric? Does it matter what you call it if it's there?

Whether it is there or not, the really exciting news for our time is
that men are living long enough for the questions to be asked. Still
outlived by women, there are, nonetheless, an impressive 20,000,000
men aged forty-five to sixty-four compared with 22,000,000 women of
that age in the United States—an increase of 15 per cent since the
1960 census of persons in this age bracket! If you include ages forty
to sixty, there are over 25,000,000 men.[1] And in the future the percentage of the total population will grow from the present 21 per
cent (aged forty-five to sixty-four) to much greater by the end of the
century.

Whatever problems men and the women who must deal with them
have in mid-life, they are relatively nothing compared to the fact
that in the past the issues were neatly dealt with by early mortality.
Middle-aged women today face increasing amounts of divorce or life
with retired husbands, the replacement for widowhood.

As far back as the 1930s, the noted anthropologist Ruth Benedict called attention to a phenomenon she called "the discontinuity of cultural conditioning" in an effort to explain the particular difficulties men face in American culture. The very cultural expectations of male superiority, responsibility, dominance, independence, and all the other attributes of a culture that placed high value on dominant masculinity, were in sharp conflict with the fact that boys were raised primarily by mothers at home and female school teachers in ordered, semiregimented school environments away from the world of work and male activity, and then cast out with minimal preparation to assume the responsibility of their assigned male roles in society. That they were often unequal to the task, faltered in "finding" themselves, and were in greater difficulty than the females of the society—raised as girls by women and making a more orderly transition to the world of dependent female roles which were more in keeping with the way in which they had been raised—did not seem surprising.[2]

It sometimes comes as a rude shock to women to realize that in such a world, becoming "male" should be more difficult than becoming "female," especially since the world seemed to value maleness so much more. Today, among women moving into roles formerly reserved for men, there is growing recognition that a world of competition, demanding technical skill, and the ability to be responsible for self and others presents similar difficulties to those faced by men.

There is still a strong tendency in this culture to believe that once a man had reached the husband-father status and had achieved his job position, whether as employee, employer, career or professional ladder, he was where he should be—the mature personality, the protecting, responsible head of household, unchanging till retirement parted him from job, or death from family and friends. Notions of personality change, career change, divorce, and life-style change, which are increasingly common among middle-aged men, still appear somewhat threatening in the light of this traditional concept of the stable, dependable, supportive male. Is there something at mid-life that precipitates a crisis for males?

Obviously, for men there is no fairly clear event or series of events equivalent to the cessation of menses for women. Males do not menstruate, males therefore have no menopause. But males, equally human, are subject to the processes of maturation and decline that accompany us from birth through our life span. The endocrine changes that affect male sexuality and aging do not suddenly occur at any one age. From about the age of thirty—the age varies depending in part probably at the particular rate of maturation of the individual—there is a gradual decline in production of male sex hormones. Male hormones (androgens) are produced by the endocrine glands. These are stimulated to produce testosterone and other male hormones by gonadatropines coming from the pituitary gland, which is, in turn, controlled by the hypothalamus, an area of the brain.[3] Shifts in the balance of sex hormones have been suggested to explain heart attacks among men.

The production of sperm also decreases as men grow older. It has been estimated that the sperm count at age seventy is about one-third that of men at age thirty-five. This in itself has no relation to the amount of sex activity or desire, and men can father children long past the age of seventy, given good health and the opportunity to do so. Men of the Caucasus, in Soviet Georgia, are known to marry late and to father children past the age of ninety! The noted Soviet gerontologist, P. A. Alikeshiev, who did much work among the people of the Caucasus, cites a case that offers a note of optimism for all men and women. He reports on one man of Daghestan who married for the third time when he was ninety. He had thirteen children by this marriage, and his wife was reported to be very pleased![4]

By their late forties and fifties, nonetheless, the signs of physical aging do become apparent even to the most robust of men—the hair a bit thinner and tinged with gray, the strength and vigor less consistent, the weight easier to put on and harder to take off, the long-distance running and championship athletics better left to younger men. In addition, and somewhat frightening, come the signs of change in body functions, increasing incidence of urinary difficulties, prostate problems, arthritis, heart conditions, and perhaps most psychologically distressing, changes in sexual functioning.

It is impossible to know, now, given the present state of knowledge, whether or not the hormonal changes occurring in males reach a critical stage in middle age, precipitating a male "menopausal syndrome," which includes depression, anxiety, irritability, fatigue, and inexplicable behavior such as giving up responsibility, searching for new life styles, women, etc. The interplay between the hormones and the psychology of the individual is still too imperfectly understood.[5] Still there is ample evidence from our culture to indicate that there are many social reasons for this period of life to be fraught with difficulty for some men, in the Western world particularly. But the experience of other men in this and other cultures does not point to the inevitability of difficulty.

First, the matter of sex. Men in our society are just as traumatized in many ways as are women by the youth cult emphasis. Sex in later life has been presented as unimportant, even non-existent. Just as it is difficult for children to accept the fact of their parents' copulation, so this is a society in which the young do not think of the old as sexual. The concept of "dirty old man" as a description of older men interested in sex is impossible to conceive of among the people of the Caucasus, for whom sexuality, albeit in moderation as are all things in their culture, is considered natural and correct. Even in our own society, to a fifty-year-old man, a forty-year-old is a vigorous youngster; to a sixty-year-old, a fifty-year-old is known to have plenty of good years left; and as far as a seventy-year-old is concerned, a man once said for his generation, "I'm still alive, aren't I?"

Masters and Johnson have again performed the service of documenting the sexual potential of men at mid-life and beyond. Yet the slightest evidence of decline of physical vigor throws some men into a state of panic, and in a sense, a self-fulfilling prophecy can go to work—expectation of loss of sexual ability can create loss of ability. There also exists a mythology believed by some that the less sex, the longer will be the ability to continue to engage in sex—a myth that runs contrary to the Masters and Johnson findings and the experience of the people of the Caucasus that continued practice with a co-operative partner is probably the best insurance for a long sex life.

Older men are different from young men in that it takes relatively longer (measured in seconds or minutes) for them to be aroused, they can maintain their erections for longer periods of time, ejaculations, therefore, come later and sexual tension is relieved less quickly —these very conditions likely to make men superior lovers. Unless there is physical illness or serious mental depression, inability to be aroused or to reach orgasm is generally a temporary condition—tied to fatigue or stress. Still, some men panic. For a wife, this can present some problems. Men seek to reassure themselves of their sexual attractiveness and ability sometimes by searching out other women, or blaming their wives for not being "sexy" enough, or they can retreat from sexuality altogether, developing functional impotence.

Yet sex at middle age and beyond is fulfilling, even better in some ways than at younger ages.

Not all men feel the need to go through life on the ready, like the proverbial jack rabbit or sexual athlete. There is a story about a seventy-year-old widower who married a beautiful twenty-five-year-old. After a few months of marriage, the young wife discovered her husband in bed with a sixty-five-year-old woman. In disbelief she asked, "What does she have that I don't?" Her husband replied, "Patience!" A frequency of intercourse several times a month to one or two times a night can prove as satisfying as the potential feat of six in succession of the seventeen-year-old. Mature sex provides the satisfactions of prolonged intimacy, joy in the warmth and togetherness of a couple. The satisfactions for a man can become diffuse, and frequent orgasm less important. Many a wife has found her middle-aged husband a far better lover than he was when young and his needs urgent.

For a few men, there is a condition known as primary testicular insufficiency. This involves failure of the testes to function, thus creating true impotence. This can be called the male climacteric, not quite equivalent to menopause—with the end of ovarian function female sexuality *does* continue. Primary testicular insufficiency is not the ordinary course for middle-aged men. Once assured that their sex lives don't end at forty or fifty or even sixty or beyond, with continued interest, opportunity, and health, men go on and on.

But life must eventually come to an end. The realization of that causes many to panic. Shakespeare wrote on the fear of death:

*Cowards die many times before their deaths;*
*The valiant never taste of death but once.*
*Of all the wonders that I yet have heard,*
*It seems to me most strange, that men should fear; Seeing that death, a*
*  necessary end,*
*Will come when it will come.*

William Shakespeare
*Julius Caesar*, Act II, Scene II

Death and taxes are indeed inevitable. Yet while we are young, there is a tendency to act as if we can "beat the system." Taxes we get used to; death, except for those of us who experience ill-timed tragedies, seems remote. But the man of forty and older has to begin to confront the fact of his mortality—he meets an old friend and they speak of mutual acquaintances—someone is bound to have had a heart attack. He reads the obituaries and there are notices of deaths of his contemporaries. He attends annual conventions, reunions, to find familiar male faces missing. Death in one's parental generation brings the inevitability closer, but the deaths of those his age bring the reality uncomfortably near.

The noted sociologist Bernice Neugarten talks about the changes that occur in the middle-aged when instead of counting "time since birth" people begin thinking in terms of "time yet to live."[6] This shift and this confrontation with the inevitability and reality of one's limited time on earth can precipitate a number of reactions. Some are terribly depressed by their awareness. I know one man who, when with friends, takes out old photos, tells stories, and recounts, "He's gone, he's finished, he's dead." His guests don't know whether to laugh or cry.

Not every man is depressed by the realization of mortality. Reggie Williams, who by the age of forty-nine had built his citizen-band radio Xtal Corporation into a multimillion-dollar industry within three years, tells of the encounter with possible death of his friends and himself at this age:

I had a scare last July. I had been to the cassette and electronic show in Chicago; we had written $12 million in orders, and I was really bushed. My neighbor was having open-heart surgery, and one of my friends in Dallas had a heart attack while driving and totaled his car, so I was kind of frightened, too. I told my wife, "Maybe you better make arrangements so that I can have a physical."[7]

The medical examination revealed that Williams was suffering from a serious heart condition which did require open-heart surgery too. Despite the frightening experience with serious illness—the operation proved to be successful—and difficulties with his seventeen-year-old son, life hasn't changed very much for him:

And now I'm back on the merry-go-round. Working harder. Longer hours. Traveling more. More stress. More strain. That is just what I shouldn't be doing after open-heart surgery. But it doesn't seem to be affecting me. I stop every once in a while and say, "Why am I pushing myself so hard?" And I say, "Why *not?* I feel great."[8]

Another reaction to mid-life is to search for ways to live one's life in the ways one had hoped to or dreamed or fantasized about. The postponements made in the past cannot be held off much longer. As one writer has said, ". . . the past floats by in a fog of hopes not realized, opportunities not grasped, women not bedded, potentials not fulfilled, and the future is a confrontation with one's own mortality."[9]

Men are not alone in this confrontation with mortality—women share the experience as well, both directly themselves, and indirectly through their husbands' and lovers' reactions. Men are particularly vulnerable, however, because of their realistic awareness of mortality statistics. They know more men are prone to heart attacks at this age level, they are aware that widows abound more than widowers, and their cultural expectations for achievement and experience have traditionally been greater than that for women.

Is there then a mid-life crisis experienced by men that precipitates personality change, different behavior, and peculiar difficulties? Are there particular cultural events that compound the realities of hormonal change and confrontation with mortality to create special problems?

In an excellent examination of the evidence by Orville G. Brim, Jr., several characteristics of American society are viewed as relevant to this question. Among them are Aspiration and Achievements, Resurgence of "The Dream," Stagnation vs. "Generativity," Relationships within the Family, Social Status and Role Changes.[10]

This is a society that places great emphasis upon personal achievement. Except for some populations, including some American Indian groups such as the Hopi, our culture encourages upward mobility, men are encouraged to do better than their fathers, and better as they grow older themselves. Education has been touted not for intellectual, aesthetic satisfactions, but rather for improved economic opportunity. As Brim states:

> Over the course of the working life, from entry to the mid-life period, it is likely that although aspirations may be adjusted downward on occasion, one usually believes there is enough time left for the desired level of achievement to be reached in future years. But during mid-life most American males must adjust their career aspirations of earlier years downward to fit current reality.[11]

For some men, the awakening, during mid-life, from the promise of this American dream can be rude and shocking and disappointing.

It would appear, though, that most men make gradual adjustments to the reality of the limitations on achievement. Americans are perhaps more vulnerable than peoples of more class-conscious traditions, where class status and limited aspirations were accepted. It would seem that psychologically it is less of a burden to be born into a socioeconomic position which is accepted, than to live in a society with the Calvinist tradition of being responsible for one's achievement and, since great value is given to achievement, feeling personal responsibility for not "making it."

There are many peoples in the world who have long shared this view of individual upward mobility as desirable, among them the Ibo of Nigeria. Others, like the Eskimo and other American Indian peoples did not particularly value this view of life in their traditions. Europeans use terms like "ambition" to describe their drive to achieve. Some men pay a price for this, particularly at mid-life. Having accepted the value system, the failure to reach the ideal—the aspiration-achievement gap—can be troublesome.

Whether or not a man is thrown into a mid-life "crisis" as a result of this confrontation with reality probably depends on how strongly his self-image is tied to the drive for economic and social success, as well as other factors.

Yet there are some men who have achieved what they set out to do, are successful in the eyes of friends, family, and society in general and still experience profound dissatisfaction at mid-life. Part of this has to do with the difficulties of maintaining one's position. Even at the top of the corporate ladders in America, men find their company ownership and executive personnel changing and must continue the struggle just to hold on to what they have. Enforced retirement at mid-life, loss of job, and economic inflation require a downward adjustment of job, position, and sometimes living standards at a time when most had anticipated the zenith of their careers. Where does one go and where does one turn when the years ahead seem to be numbered? For the man in early-middle age—with more time—the problem is, of course, somewhat different from that of the man in late-middle age.

Work remains a major part of life for American men during middle age. The facts indicate that between the ages of forty-five and fifty-four, 93 per cent of men are in the labor force. Between fifty-five and sixty-four the percentage drops to 81 per cent and after that falls off precipitously. This compares with 54 per cent of women aged forty-five to fifty-four and 42 per cent of those aged fifty-five to sixty-four. But men, unlike women, are less represented in the labor force at ages forty-five to sixty-four (an average of 87 per cent) than are younger men aged twenty-five to forty-four, 94 per cent of whom are in the labor force.[12]

Holding on to one's work, whether because of the pleasure, status, or fulfillment of values it provides or because of necessity, is increasingly more difficult as one grows older. For some men, the loss of position and the transition to retirement, whether voluntary or enforced, can be a difficult adjustment to make.

But what of the man who suffers middle-age malaise even though he has achieved what he set out to do and is relatively secure in his position? Brim speaks of "The Dream" as a youthful aspiration, as an early image of the future self which never dies. Despite his achievement, Brim argues,

> The man may feel that he has attempted too little, not stretched himself, not seized opportunities. He may feel it is meaningless and ask, is this what I really wanted? Was it worth all I had to give up? Do I want to go on doing these things for the years I have left? What of those parts of myself that I had to neglect—to suppress—to sacrifice? There is a pervading sense of sadness in these mid-life men of unfulfilled dreams.[13]

The process of resolution of this crisis can be astonishing to some wives, who find their husbands ready to throw off accustomed behavior, career, family, in the search for the life of their dreams, or who find their husbands or lovers plunged into a state of melancholy.

I would suggest that it is not only the resurgence of youthful dreams that contributes to this problem. Middle-aged men are also subject to the stimulation and examples of the current world. An achieved goal which seemed desirable a generation ago, may seem trivial in the present, for one's sons and their contemporaries are defining their lives in even more far-reaching terms than their fathers. Unlike the traditional Eskimos who aspired to be *as good* as their fathers, our sons are expected to aim far higher. One is reminded of the teasing ad for a top brand of Scotch which goes like this, "Your son has just bought the most expensive hi-fi equipment on the market and you're still drinking *that* cheap brand." A man might be grateful for having achieved the ability to purchase what he wants, but the ad taunts. It is as if in a society that stresses constant achievement, the dreams of one's youth and the changing present make it impossible to win. There seems to be an urgency at mid-life for a man to re-evaluate who he is, what he has been doing, and where he wants to go—to start all over on another rung of the ladder.

There is also the possibility in mid-life that some men require the sense of continued growth—that they resist deeply the possibility of stagnation and degeneration. Psychoanalyst Erik Erikson has suggested that one adult task is the resolution of stagnation vs. generativity. For him, the successful resolution is the older generation's acceptance of its responsibility to care for the next generation. Brim suggests, ". . . a desire for a sense of personal growth is a deep-seated characteristic of the human organism and that a failure of a sense of growth generates depression and leads to attempts to avoid this stagnation."[14]

In this culture, when men are taught to believe that life is pretty much over by the end of middle age, the fear of stagnation may be very intense. Contrast this with cultures, such as among the Australian aborigines, in which older men are the repositories of the wisdom and knowledge of the tribe, and with cultures where the older are the closer to the spirit world and thus worthy of greater respect and admiration. To be "finished," a "has been," can come relatively early in the life of American males, especially to those who have reached a high level of success early in their youth. Competition seems to level off in middle age in all societies, where men leave the more vigorous competitive tasks to the younger.[15] But our society offers few rewards for a withdrawal from competition either in the business or political or sports arenas, the traditional stamping grounds of men. In social life, the leisure of retirement requires adjustment to unaccustomed roles. In contrast, many traditional societies, especially those preliterate, invest their aging men with the powers befitting their experience and wisdom.

Men, like women, also face a period of considerable change in their family relationships during the period of mid-life: children growing, leaving home, sometimes providing great joy, at other times enormous disappointment; elderly parents ill and dying, frequently financially and emotionally dependent; wives also experiencing the passing years. And then there is the single scene, for those men who

have left their marriages in the search for a better life, or the need to
do their own thing, responding in part to the call of the popular culture illustrated by the popular song lyrics dealing with *having* to be
me or *having* to be free or *having* to do it my way—often to find it
little better than what they left behind.

Despite the fact that the mass media and the popular culture seem
to be beckoning men to the single life, it is interesting to note that
according to the last census 85 per cent of the men forty-five to sixty-
four were married, compared with 73 per cent of the women that
age. And it is also true, despite what their fantasies might be, men
were not dashing off to marry young women. Only some 2.9 per cent
of men aged forty-five to fifty-four were married to women under the
age of thirty-four. The vast majority of men, 60.3 per cent, were married to women forty-five to fifty-four; and less than one third were
married to women aged thirty-five to forty-four. Pretty much the
same situation exists for men in later middle age. Ninety-one per cent
of all married men aged fifty-five to sixty-four were married to
women between the ages of forty-five to sixty-four. And within both
categories of early and late middle-aged men, 5 per cent of the marriages were with women older than themselves.[16]

In general, in this society, men tend to marry women younger
than themselves, but only slightly younger, most marriages occurring
between men and women within a ten-year age span. The wives of
middle-aged men are likely to be very close to or middle-aged themselves.

Most unmarried men aged forty-five to sixty-four are either divorced, separated, or were never married. Only 3 per cent are widowed, compared with 13 per cent of the women who are widowed.
This might seem like further evidence of how fragile life is for males
—but it must be remembered that women are married to older men,
and this affects the mortality statistics. It also reflects the continuing
tendency for men to marry and live in family groups—most men do
not remain bachelors.

Curiously enough, an American wife is likely to find her middle-
aged husband more dependent, more domestic, more in need of
affection and support than ever before. At the same time, middle-
aged wives may be more independent than in earlier stages of
their marriage. They are likely to be providing greater nurturance to
sons, daughters, and grandchildren and elderly parents or moving out

of the home into career or community activity at a time when their husbands are requiring more of them. Some wives find that the time, attention, and companionship they craved early in their marriages— but were not available because of a husband's attention to career and friends—become available at a time when they have grown unaccustomed to them and have found other interests and time-consuming activities. How a wife reacts to her husband's new requirements must have some effects on the men at mid-life. I am reminded of a letter to the advice column of a daily newspaper. It read: "I married my husband for better or worse, but not for lunch. Now that he's retired I have no time with my friends." The answer was to the point. "If you don't have lunch with him, he'll find someone else who will."

Growing independence of the wife has been suggested as a major source of problems for some middle-aged men, who fear the loss of a primary source of recognition, affection, and sense of value at the very time in their lives when these are no longer provided by job and outside interests.

Clearly, middle age is a time when various changes or transitions can be anticipated: children leaving home, parents ill or dying, job changes. Some of these events are unhappy, stressful occurrences. Others are not necessarily so. Job change or retirement, becoming a grandparent, can bring new pleasures, and more and more evidence indicates that couples report greater happiness after their children leave home.

In her extensive and fascinating work on middle age, Bernice Neugarten has called attention to the phenomenon of "on-time and off-time." Her hypothesis is that most of us are pretty well socialized into expecting life to change and events to occur throughout our lifetimes. The stressful events are those that occur at times when they were unanticipated:

> . . . it is the unanticipated, not the anticipated, which is likely to represent the traumatic event. Major stresses are caused by events that upset the sequence and rhythm of the expected life cycle, as when death of a parent comes in adolescence rather than in middle age; when the birth of a child is too early or too late; when occupational achievement is delayed; when the empty nest, grandparenthood, retirement, major illness, or widowhood occur off-time.[17]

The experience of a man at middle age is also shared in part with the others of his generation. Over one half of the men aged forty-five to sixty-four, for example, in the United States are veterans of World War II. Among those aged forty-five to fifty-four, over 72 per cent are veterans. For some men that war experience was profoundly traumatic; for others it was the high point of their lives. Joseph Heller, who vividly described the shenanigans of the young men of World War II in his popular *Catch 22*, describes the malaise and disappointment for his older protagonist in the more recent novel *Something Happened.*[18]

The generation that experienced the great depression of the 1930s came to mid-life with a different perspective from that of their sons, who lived with the youth culture of the 1960s, the Viet Nam War, Watergate, and the sexual revolution. And what of the millions of people at one time or another in history who leave their roots, cross oceans and continents, move from farm to city, and forge new lives in new places? Some are the first to make the changes; others are born with the adjustments already begun by parents. In any generation there will have been a wide variety of experience, but major events such as world wars, or holocausts must affect some generations differently from that of others.

There is one group of males in the cosmopolitan world for whom growing older presents some special problems—the world of the homosexuals. To be "gay" in itself creates difficulties in relation to the "straight" world, especially where definitions of illegality intrude on the sexual privacy and economic life of the gay male. But within the gay world itself, middle-age can exacerbate the difficulties of achieving desired relationships and satisfactions, exaggerating the problems sometimes faced by normal heterosexual men.

Middle age comes early for homosexuals. *Beauty*, physical beauty, is a prime concern in the relationships between gays. Relationships are frequently brief and are primarily for the physical pleasure they provide. Therefore, the body is critical. Younger homosexuals regard men of thirty as "over the hill." And, since many gays live very intense lives, conducive to dissipation, an early decline of the physical body is not unusual.

But, as in the heterosexual world, not all people are ever the same; older men who are experienced lovers as well as cultivated, interesting persons retain interest from more intelligent gays. And, as in the straight world, older men with money have greater access to younger, attractive men who use the relationship to their economic advantage. On the other hand, many middle-aged gay couples lead conservative lives which include intimacy, friendship, love, and responsibility for one another.

Because homosexuality has not been taken very seriously by social scientists until recently, there is little data to tell us just how age relationships are actually distributed, but interviews with homosexuals suggest that physical beauty in a partner remains of primary concern in sexual relationships for older gays. Young gays who have relationships with both younger and older men tend to separate out sex with the young and beautiful from friendships and emotional attachments to middle-aged gays. But there is hardly a conversation with a homosexual without some reference to abhorrence of the body in decline.

Middle-aged gays of today have also known a social experience with their homosexuality somewhat different from that of younger people. The experience for some has been more difficult. They were young homosexuals at a time when they were required to be more furtive, hiding their inclinations, being the "closet queens." Younger gays have had a different experience, becoming gays in a time when there was public acknowledgment, greater tolerance of their status, and community in the "gay liberation" movement. There is then a sort of generation gap between those coming of age after World War II and earlier generations. Younger gays find less in common with the older generation because of their history of concealment, furtiveness, etc. But, as in the straight world, the older people who have cultivated their minds and sensibilities retain interest for each other, attract younger people, and appear to have fewer problems with their aging. And, whether it be mid-life crisis or simply a matter of keeping up with the times, increasing numbers of middle-aged gays have been "coming out of the closet," declaring themselves, leaving heterosexual marriages, and living openly in the gay world.

There also appears to be a generation gap as regards homosexual sex roles. Young gays I have talked with who have had considerable sexual experience say that older gays seem to be more rigid as regards their acting of sex roles, some "give," others "receive," i.e., some are active playing the "male" role and others passive, playing the "female" role. Among younger gays the giving and receiving are interchangeable—there is greater spontaneity in the sex act. Thus, middle-aged lovers are not as desirable to younger ones who have participated in what might be called the gay version of the sexual revolution—or "out from under."

Yet, middle age among gays is not simply a matter of pessimistic disadvantage, characterized by loss of youth and beauty, and by the closet-queen experience and rigid sex roles. There are some real advantages which come with advancing age, and which are appreciated by the sensitive and intelligent. Despite their aging bodies they can be more experienced and skillful lovers. Capable of more courtship time, and able to maintain erections for longer times, they are less of the "slam bang, thank you ma'am (sir?)" kind of casual encounter. Also, if interesting, cultivated persons when young, how much more so after years of continued cultivation, learning, and experience? Perhaps most important, the older homosexual who has achieved self-acceptance, maturity, has a potential for being far less troubled than a younger man, and these attributes lend to him an air of attractiveness.

For young gays, becoming middle-aged is a reality they must deal with. One young man told me, "I am developing my talents and abilities so that I won't be totally dependent on youth and beauty in my relationships with others."

Despite their own minority status in the population, and despite their own experience with prejudice and what they regard as abuse and unfair treatment, male homosexuals continue to share the larger society's views of older women. There are always some women who enjoy the company of gays, whether it is because of the fact that they are non-aggressive or "safe" sexually, or because they are artistic or whatever. Among gays these women are frequently referred to when young as "fruit flies." Older women are called "fag hags"!

The gay liberation movement has not been without its problems for women. Encouragement to reject the closet-queen life has led many out of heterosexual marriages, some of which were long standing and included grown children.

I know of a woman who had been married some twenty-five years to the same man, and had two grown children. For nearly the last ten years of her marriage, she had had practically no intercourse with her husband. He berated her for being unstimulating, and inadequate in bed. She believed herself frigid, and with her husband's encouragement had been undergoing psychiatric treatment in an attempt to be a responsive, stimulating wife. Naïvely convinced of her blame for the poor sex life within her marriage, it never occurred to her that the fault lay elsewhere. What a shock to her when her husband declared himself tired of his closet-queen existence and left her for the male lover he had known for many years!

The greater acceptance of homosexuality in some cosmopolitan situations has also made it possible for those who had suppressed homosexual leanings to move out into the welcoming gay world. The sexual revolution which encouraged greater spontaneity in sexual behavior has affected not only relationships between men and women, but the freer expression of sexuality by latent homosexuals. For a thoroughly heterosexual wife, a middle-age transition to the gay world by her husband can be a profoundly shocking event. It is difficult enough for a woman when her husband leaves for another woman, but to leave her for a man?

It is obvious, then, that middle age presents special problems for men as it does for women. But it is far from clear that a mid-life crisis is inevitable or that men suffer a "menopausal" syndrome, including depression, anxiety, irritability, fatigue, etc.

There is no marked biological event; hormonal changes are gradual and occur over a long period of time. There is no clear evidence that male hormonal changes precipitate emotional crises for men. Men in this culture retain certain advantages over women in that their attractiveness is not as directly associated with youth as for women— tinges of gray are "distinguished," the robust thickened body is "masculine," wrinkles about the eyes are "laugh" lines, and not only younger women are available, but also a skewed sex ratio in later years means that for every available male there are likely to be female partners waiting in the wings—some one hundred women for every ninety-one males at ages forty-five to sixty-four.

At the same time, there are no clear-cut cultural events that necessarily precipitate men into a mid-life crisis. Many of the events that occur, and which have been described, are not necessarily unhappy ones, nor stressful enough to precipitate crisis.

Yet, some men do suffer depression in their mid-life, and this depression is probably the fundamental symptom of mid-life crisis when it does occur. True psychological depression is somewhat different from ordinary grief or sadness which can be readily ex-

plained by some precipitating factor such as a death, loss of job, etc.
In true depression there is an involuntary relatively incapacitating
sense of worthlessness and hopelessness, or deep fatigue and other
physical complaints. Some men, like women, turn to alcohol, withdraw socially, and may become impotent. Others turn to philandering, womanizing, in an effort to demonstrate their vigor.

However, depression is not limited to mid-life—most middle-aged
males are not depressed—and alcoholism in the United States is not
limited to persons in mid-life!

Cross-cultural evidence would also seem to support the view that a
mid-life crisis is not inevitable for men. Margaret Mead, the noted
anthropologist, has been quoted as saying:

> I would expect to find depression among late-middle-aged men in
> societies where the diminutions of aging, such as the loss of strength
> are important. But, if old age means having wisdom and skills that
> don't require physical strength, that's fine. The Australian aboriginal
> men, when they grow older, had all the ceremonial wisdom and so got
> most of the younger women, and it isn't reported to have depressed
> them.[19]

Among many peoples of the world, middle age, instead of toppling a
man from the heights of his achievement, moves him into positions
of greater authority, power, and wealth.

There is no simple answer to the question of why some men in
modern American society find the mid-life period one of greater crisis than do other men, although it is clear that during mid-life there
are transitions that have to be made, and any such period is likely to
be stressful. Probably, as for women, mid-life is a particularly vulnerable time because of the many social factors described above. For
some men the stresses may come too close together, and they may experience events more intensely than do other men. Experiencing divorce or the serious illness or death of a wife, the death of parents,
the loss or change of job, the leaving of children all within a brief
span of time can precipitate the sense of mid-life crisis.

And again, the confrontation with one's own mortality probably is
experienced by men with greater vividness than for women. Women
also recognize that now one must think of the "time yet to live," but
for men the reality of death makes that time seem uncomfortably
short.

How a particular man responds to his mid-life experiences is of course difficult to predict. Middle age now extends over some twenty years. The stressful events of this period may be distributed throughout this time, or they may be clustered together within a brief interval. A man brings to his experiences a previous life history, expectations, state of health, and an individual set of relationships with others. There does not seem to be any inevitable progression or series of personality changes in this life period. And the potential for contentment and happiness and the capacity to love and enjoy life remains.

While there is, however, the common cultural expectation that women will have problems in middle age, still, as the anonymous letter to the editor quoted at the beginning of this chapter implies, there is a tendency for men to suppress their discomforts with growing older.

In her perceptive article, "Is There a Male Menopause?", Martha Weinman Lear describes a poignant letter to the editors of *Medical Economics*. In it a physician's wife writes that her husband was showing all the symptoms of what she assumed to be the male menopausal syndrome. He was depressed, had lost interest in his practice, all sexual interest in her, and she loved him very much and was worried. The advice from the editors describe her husband as either suffering from the Gauguin syndrome (Gauguin being the French painter who left Paris behind for life on Tahiti in the South Seas), the Scapegoat Wife syndrome (in which the wife is blamed for the man's problems), or the Sacred Amulet syndrome (in which declining sexual powers are believed to be magically restored extramaritally). They recommended psychiatric treatment for her husband's condition. The prognosis was good, they believed he would be cured in a year.

A plethora of letters to the editor followed the publication of the letter and the advice. Almost to a man, the writers agreed that the primary cause of the "Medical Man's Menopause" was neither his hormones nor his neuroses nor his environment but, in fact, his wife![20]

IV

# The Beauty Industry — Friend or Enemy?

There are exquisite beaches on the isles of the sunny Aegean, where, in the sultry afternoons, there lie an array of stunning nudes. Covered with only an assortment of oils, lotions, and creams, to coax their skins to a uniform bronze glow, it is impossible to tell a former queen from a shopkeeper's assistant, the bright from the dull, the educated from the illiterate, the French from the German, the American from the Swede. Their system for placing one another into some system for recognition cuts through all class and ethnic barriers—they will ask: "What sign are you?" It is through the use of astrological signs that they determine who are what, using astrology as a neutral way of communicating with persons, who in their workaday real worlds they would have no reason or even willingness to be with.

Mankind everywhere makes some effort to define social situations and to place people within them in such a way that the appropriate kinds of behavior can be expressed. But what is considered correct and appropriate varies from place to place. What was appropriate a generation ago may be inappropriate now, and the same behavior can mean many different things to different people.

On those beaches in Greece, nudism is ordinary, uneventful, and accepted. Not so at Miami Beach or Atlantic City. A strong handshake and straightforward look in the eye are signs of trust and good character in most of Western society. Among the Chomula of Mexico, as among many other peoples, a straightforward look in the eye means just the opposite, marking one as a suspicious character. And for many people a strong handshake, rather than representing hearty good fellowship, as among Americans, is sometimes regarded as an intrusion on a person's private body space.

And what is considered the appropriate behavior and appearance of middle-aged women is very much the result of what the society and time in which they live believes to be the case.

Our society places so much stress on youth and good looks that women are justifiably concerned with the passing years and the toll they take on appearance. Women find themselves in a bind. On the one hand, they must make great efforts to remain attractive in order to retain social and sexual acceptability and to remain active in the world of work and politics. On the other hand, they are often chided for refusing to accept the "natural" beauty of age. It is through their appearance—far more than by their astrological signs—that women declare their readiness to be judged as active participants in life.

Attempts to belittle women's efforts to adorn themselves, to use cosmetics, hair dyes, dress, have always struck me as being rather sad. These are precisely the steps a woman takes to declare to the world that she is part of it, that she is refusing to be moved by a younger age group into a new position, that of the aged, which in our society has so little status and is considered to be a period of retirement from sexual, vocational, and even social encounters. In her novel of the middle-aged woman, discouragingly entitled *Summer Before the Dark*, Doris Lessing has her middle-aged heroine declare her independence from family and societal demands by allowing her dyed hair to grow out so that there was a broad band of gray on either side of the part.[1] Certainly, if a woman decides to allow a natural growth of gray hair, that is her decision—it is often a very becoming style— but as a declaration of independence, whether fictional or not, it does not seem to make much sense. Independence from what? From society? It seems to me that this heroine's gesture represents more an acceptance of the role imposed by the society about her that she appear as an old, less desirable, and less socially active woman, retired from the world of work and love. This is not independence, it is fulfilling a social expectation.

Grooming the body is a universal human activity. Even our primate cousins spend hours cleaning one another, caring for their appearance. Women are hardly the only ones to use cosmetics and care for their hair and skin. Masai young men in Africa spend days anointing and braiding their hair into the hundreds of braided ringlets of their elegant hairdos. The bows and ribbons and wigs of the courts of France and England, the Edwardian gentlemen, epitomized the very finest of the well-dressed gentlemen of their time. Rouged cheeks, powdered wigs, and perfume, have been used in many places and times by men as well as women. But fashions change, and in our more recent generations in the Western world, the males have, at least until very recently, been expected to provide the plain backdrop for decorative women.

Women, and men as well, have probably always adorned themselves, from the earliest beginnings of society. In the Cro-Magnon caves of Southern Europe, where men and women lived over twenty thousand years ago, there were found red ochre paint pots. We know that the ancient peoples of Sumeria, the Far East and Egypt used cosmetics widely. People everywhere have in one way or another attempted to improve on the human condition by cutting, shaving, plucking, braiding, or setting the hair; by deodorizing, anointing, perfuming, scarring the skin; by painting or stretching the lips; by cutting, sanding, painting the nails; painting the eyes and face; dyeing the skin and hair; filing the teeth, reshaping the bite; molding, developing, and concealing parts of the body.

Fashion and fad have always played a large part in choice of style, and what is appropriate in one place and time and group of people may be totally inappropriate in others.² Fashionable New Yorkers would hardly accept the filing of teeth to pointed shapes that some West African peoples admire, but almost all the stars of Broadway and television undergo arduous dentistry to get fancy caps to give their teeth a shiny, even appearance. In some places, women have surgery to shorten their noses, in others they insert plugs to lengthen them. The Mayas of ancient Yucatan used to dangle string between the eyes of their baby girls to force them to acquire what they considered to be the beautiful look of crossed eyes!

What is beautiful is largely beautiful in the eyes of the beholder— what is beautiful to some is not beautiful to others. And the things we consider beautiful are largely what we have learned to believe are beautiful. I suppose it might be argued that there could be a universal standard of beauty—but what that is, is difficult to agree upon. Perhaps one standard is health. Good health would seem to be the basis for beauty anywhere. But once the factor of health is cancelled out there remains the problem of a wide variety of cultural differences concerning what is and what is not beautiful.

The emphasis upon youth and the slender form in our culture as being the epitome of beauty misleads us into thinking of this as a universal, natural condition. The middle-age spread that so many women dread, and fight with exercise and diet, for other women represents a highly desirable appearance. For example, among Gypsy women the large person is highly admired, and the ease with which weight and size seem to increase at middle age is a matter of rejoicing, not pain as a result. The Indians of the Guatemalan highlands also admire a woman of great size. Indeed, in much of the world, girth represents prosperity and well-being among people who struggle for enough to eat, and is not easily deprecated. And among ourselves just over one hundred years ago, the great beauty and actress Sarah Bernhardt was described: "Whenever Mme. Sarah comes over to America, she looks fatter and fairer and absolutely younger . . ."[3]

But the fact is that we do live within our own culture—now. Being big and heavy is not a necessary condition of middle age, is not necessarily healthy—can, on the contrary, be decidedly unhealthy—and we also know that being heavy is not admired. Women who make an effort to keep their bodies in good physical condition, who work at exercise to stay shapely as well as to maintain tone and good circulation, who watch their diets, stay away from a life of overindulgence or dissipation really deserve much admiration. Their refusal to fulfill any expectation that "they go to pot" is a statement of independence, precisely the opposite of what much of society tries to impose upon women as they grow older.

The women who say, "It doesn't matter," are really, in a sense, giving in. It does matter, because it is a declaration of belonging. And our society does much disservice to women when it persists in labeling efforts to retain a youthful body as somehow inappropriate or even obscene.

Women's magazines have always been somewhat ambivalent in their approach to women in this regard. On the one hand, their pages have been filled with commendable advice on how to keep a marvelous figure, but on the other hand, their pages have been filled with photos of absolutely emaciated young girls who were supposed to represent the model toward which one should aspire. Fortunately, in more recent years, the pages of *Harper's* and *Vogue* and other leading magazines have begun to portray stunning women in their forties and fifties in their feature articles—but the photographers' models stay the age of their daughters. Nonetheless, a generation of women educated by fashion magazines, even if they are realistic about their not being stunning, are not about to give in simply because it takes a little more effort to keep good body tone the older one gets. And for that the magazines really should be thanked. The sedentary lives most urban industrialized people live require this special attention to the body. Women who work on farms, or who were busy gathering food or walking long distances daily to fetch water and wood didn't need the expertise of the exercise salon. Their way of life, as the way of life of most women throughout history, provided the activity to maintain good body tone and circulation. Modern women must work at this, or play as the case may be, via sport and gymnastics, swimming, and dance.

But what of the hair, the skin, the use of cosmetics to smooth the wrinkle, hide the faded look? Are cosmetics and dress merely the frivolities of the idle rich, the very young? Are women merely the victims of the multimillion dollar grooming industry promising us the illusion of youth and beauty, denying us the "natural" beauty of age?

So often, older women get the message that they should "look your age," to dress in ways considered proper for members of their generation. They are teased and laughed at for "dressing like a teenager." People speak of the "Palm Beach syndrome," referring to women of a certain age dressing and making up like young women. Sometimes this attitude toward older women is expressed in pretty astonishing ways. I remember one woman's encounter while shopping and her first realization that she was not as young as she had been. As a young woman, what seemed to be older saleswomen would at times honestly say, "This dress doesn't do a thing for you." But the years did pass and there came a day when a very young salesgirl smirked, "You don't do a thing for this dress."

As far as dressing your age is concerned, a look about the world tells us how capricious are the ways of fashion, and how seemingly arbitrary are the choices of symbols to tell age. The dress with the deep decolletage is considered fine for the young, while the older woman is so often encouraged to wear the turtle neck, or high-necked dress with scarf to hide flesh and wrinkles. But in Africa, it is the oldest women who still carry their burdens proudly on their heads above their bare torsos, breasts exposed, while their young, fashionable daughters, educated in mission and government schools, cover their bodies. Blue jeans and slacks were the "in" look for young women in the 1960s. But old Chinese women have known the comfort of trousers for centuries.

In our own experience, when middle-aged women took to their

pant suits in the 1970s, their daughters suddenly rediscovered dresses and high heels; when older women raised their hems during the mini-skirt craze, down came the hems and the midi-skirt was now a hit, considered high style rather than middle-aged dowdy.

Still, middle-aged women do have the fashion industry with its mass-production facilities and advertising to thank for helping them in what seems to be the difficult battle to "stay with it." I realize that the industry is often blamed for its apparent unreasonable swings in fashion, creating budget crises over seemingly useless wardrobes, great last year, impossible to wear this time around. And there are, certainly, justifiable complaints one can raise about their choice of cut and color and bewildering variety creating confusion and expense for women generally. But, on balance, it seems that they have helped women rather than hurt. This generation of women, in the modern industrialized nations, has available to it, in remarkably short time, clothing in all price ranges and all sizes and shapes duplicating the accepted symbols of fashionable dress—and to be fashionable is to declare to the people around that one is very much a part of the mainstream of society. It is a presentation of self that declares desire to be a participant in life.

It is a mistake, an oversimplification, to attribute to a woman's desire to be fashionable only the motive of insecurity and wanting to go along as a conformist. Certainly there are many women for whom being dressed fashionably is important mainly because they *require* the symbols of dress to feel comfortable in social situations. Knowing that people think you look good, or even beautiful, can provide a boost toward making a woman feel at ease. But dress alone will hardly counteract any basic personality or intellectual incapacity. The eighteenth-century feminist Mary Wollstonecraft noted this when she wrote in *A Vindication of the Rights of Women*, ". . . weak are the women who imagine that they can long please without the aid of the mind, . . ."[4] And there are women who are afraid to look different, who are excessively concerned with "what they're wearing."

But these women are not necessarily neurotic, and they do symbolize things that are a part of all of us: the recognition that others require some help via symbols—dress and grooming—to help them determine how to act toward us. Dress serves this function in the way that astrology does for nudists, and to be too differently attired in a social situation calls either for unnecessary attention, or brands us as socially inept. Any woman who really cares about how others will treat her knows how important are the seemingly capricious and superficial symbols of clothing and grooming. For in playing social roles women not only have to *feel* the part, they have to *look* the part as well. It could be argued that the very secure, mature woman knows who she is and doesn't need the artificial appurtenances of cloth and paint, the costume of a role, in order to "be herself." But our selves are many things. We are mothers, employees, employers, teachers, students, lovers, shoppers, housewives, hostesses. What we feel about our selves is highly significant; but, what is also significant, is how others react toward us. And appropriate responses to our many roles involve not only how we feel about ourselves but how others feel about us—and the reactions of others are affected by the way we present ourselves, by our behavior and our *appearance*.

There is, of course, a difference between being fashionably dressed and being appropriately dressed. To be appropriately dressed means that the wearer shows some understanding of the nature of the social situation in which she is.[5] For example, ordinarily it is not appropriate to wear a ball gown, complete with silver slippers and baubles, to do Saturday morning shopping at the supermarket. Sunday morning, after an all-night fiesta, might be understandable, but the lady so dressed on Saturday would draw much attention and would have to have a pretty good reason not to be considered exceedingly peculiar.

But even the matter of appropriate dress changes with the fashions. A generation ago women teachers were fired for wearing slacks; today their garb ranges all the way from maxi- to mini-skirt, with various lengths of trousers in between.

There are some women, bearing an aura of charisma, who are in the vanguard of fashion, setting the new style. Others can completely ignore fashion and still get the kinds of attention and admiration they seek. Greta Garbo could wear her pants without any difficulty at a time when they were unthinkable for the well-dressed woman and would have meant dismissal for the working woman. Anthropologist Margaret Mead with her simple garb and shepherd's crook makes a striking figure overshadowing the elegantly dressed ladies on television talk shows. But most women are not extraordinary individuals. For most, showmanship is neither easy nor successful.

While some dress is appropriate for social situations, not all dress represents good taste, and the older woman is no different from any other in the need to be concerned about using good taste in dress and grooming. The little knit dress might be just the thing to wear to the office, but if it is too little, and the bulge of flesh around the waist is made bigger than ever by the clinging fabric, that is clearly bad taste.

Many people feel that women have to be concerned about their dress and grooming because our culture requires conformity, and they resent the imposition on them. They would argue that the independent thinker should emancipate herself from the tyranny imposed by the society's demands to dress fashionably, "appropriately," and in good taste. Many of these critics would argue that our individuality is stifled as a result and to do our own thing represents a revolt against the intolerable social pressures to conform. But a look about the world, both through history and around the many cultures in it, points out how relatively non-conformist our culture actually permits us to be. We live in a world where the motto is "Junior is a size, not an age." There is room for great discretion in grooming and dress compared with other times and places. The hooded veils of Moslem women, imposed for centuries, were a *requirement* which had to be followed. For a woman to unveil herself in public, before recent years—and the requirement is still in force in many places in the mid-East—meant ostracism and even death. For many groups of Orthodox Jews, marriage imposed a *requirement* that women wear wigs—and there was no choice in the matter. The girls of Transylvania were permitted to wear so-called "pearly wreaths" on their heads *only* if they were virgins.[6] Strings about the waist, aprons, jewelry, cosmetics, and scarring, have all at one time or another been *requirements* for women of certain ages and social position in their society—the only acceptable forms of dress and grooming permitted them.

Women of the modern world have an enormous array of choices set before them, and they can exercise a wide degree of taste, discretion, and individuality.

What are the important factors that help determine the choices a woman makes? For whom, or for what does she actually dress? Surely, many women dress or groom themselves because they like to please themselves. The reflection in the mirror sends a message back, giving pleasure or disappointment. A little help to make that reflection more desirable gives the spirit a lift. For the narcissistic woman, interested only in herself, this may be the primary reason—self-satisfaction. There is a thin line between narcissism and vanity, however. The vain woman is very concerned about how she looks, and a bit of vanity helps keep her interested in her appearance. The narcissistic woman is overly involved with self, and narcissism can be a symptom of neurosis, when grooming crowds out all other aspects of living and interest in others.

Some women dress for the men in their lives—to please them, to give them high social status, or to stimulate them sexually.

To appear attractive to the man you love seems to be a pretty normal thing, yet there are so many convolutions and complications created around this very simple matter of simply appearing aesthetically satisfying, for we're back again to what we learn to judge as pleasing. For the men of traditional Greece, the married women dressed in plain black and sitting at their doorways or verandas, passing the cool evening with the womenfolk, represent the model of modesty and good taste—non-provocative to other men and provoking no scandal—the very picture of the good wife trying to please her husband. For the modern American, yes and even the modern Greek, to return home after a day at work or the office, to find a plainly garbed, "dowdy" housewife is the opposite of what all the media have taught him is an attractive woman. And her plainness and dowdiness send a message out to him as well—that he doesn't matter enough for her to have to groom and dress herself.

Feminists are justifiably annoyed with the idea that women should dress for men. Mostly, this is based upon the fact that there is an exploitative element in the relationship between some men and the women who garb themselves for them, and that in addition, some of these women are nothing except when defined in relation to these men. In our society, wealthy men, and even those not so wealthy, look upon women as adornments, as symbols of their own high positions, whether derived from money, virility, power or what have you. The beautiful woman, extremely well-groomed and well-dressed, announces to the world for him, "Look what *I* am able to have." These women, generally, are the young and extremely attractive, with the keenest of fashion sense about their bodies, clothes, and cosmetics. Many feminists, and older women as well who either cannot or will not take such a role, frequently reject this relationship to men by deliberately disdaining fashionable grooming. It seems to me that these women, while they have a right to their attitudes and life styles, are biting off their noses to spite their faces. Being well turned out does not *by itself* place any woman in an exploited relationship to men. And there are many other social reasons for appearance to have significance.

Of course, dress and grooming have their sexual aspects—women do dress to attract and stimulate men. But it would be an exaggeration to consider this the primary purpose of dress. After all, the naked body was and still is our original equipment, and the perpetuation of the species has done very nicely without the benefit of clothes. The nude remains an erotic figure. But clothing and cosmetics help the interplay among the sexes while, not so incidentally, protecting us from cold or heat, rain, and wind. A bit of covering here and there, a dash of color, an ornament or two, assembled in the ways defined by the culture as appealing, attract and titillate the senses and, accompanied by the appropriate gestures, announce availability. The woman who does not care about her looks sends out a message that she is not interested, not available. And this may be exactly the opposite of the message intended.

Those women who are concerned that the men interested in them be interested in who they are, in their minds not simply their bodies, are deluding themselves if they think that men can totally escape the aesthetic judgments imposed on their senses by their cultures. A dash of conscious attention to appearance cannot hurt these relationships.

Sociologist George Simmel, writing in the late nineteenth century, pointed out that sexuality was only one part of the function of grooming in Western society. The larger function of grooming is better understood as sociability.[7] And this makes sense when we recognize that most women, most of the time—the true narcissist is an exception—dress in anticipation of social situations. They dress for a time and place in which others will be present and, for the most part, how careful they are depends on not only their particular personalities and habits, but largely upon *who* will be present, whether her peers or social superiors, or people she is unconcerned about, does not know and will never see again, or whether she is alone.

Many housewives, when they go to work in offices or shops, find themselves dressing and grooming themselves more carefully than ever. And this at a time when they objectively have less time than ever before. Sociologist Murray Wax has pointed to the fact that these women now have an audience of male and female peers alert to their appearance. The housewife, on the other hand, may be socializing mainly by phone, unseen and isolated from men and women and, thus, more likely to "neglect her appearance." That same housewife, out to lunch with her friend is likely to dress and groom herself for that social occasion.

Women are aware of these social stimulants to grooming. A dress is bought for "an occasion," a new lipstick for the weekend holiday, the weekly shampoo and set to look good in the office, and a new outfit for a new date. A great boost to the fashion industry should come with the invention and use of a telephone-television machine. Imagine the ads—"Clothes to be seen in while talking long distance!"

There are, of course, those who would reject the standards imposed by our culture. They would argue that our standards are false, based on crass commercialism, and that they devalue the natural beauty of women. They see beauty in the wrinkled brow, years of experience and wisdom etched upon the older face. But, except for those women living in traditional ethnic situations, in which age is valued, and older women—mothers and grandmothers—venerated, this picture represents romantic nonsense for most of us. Women in the Western industrial world may not particularly value the standards that belittle their aging, and may very well wish to have these value judgments changed. Indeed, they may very actively take part in those movements, including the feminist movements, that seek to change society's attitudes toward women in general and older women in particular. But the fact remains that for most women, here and now, the current standards affect the way they are looked upon and the way they are treated!

A woman cannot help but know, from the behavior of others toward her, that the way in which she is dressed and groomed tells a great deal about her position in the society, and the way she acts in relationship to some audience of people. She knows that to appear for work in the careless array of her appearance when alone in her kitchen in the morning, won't win her a promotion, and indeed might mark her as somewhat of a "kook." And unfortunate as the case may be, to neglect the opportunities to retain a fashionable, youthful, attractive appearance will speedily increase the audience to consider her sexually unattractive, less desirable for employment, and uninteresting socially. Women cannot be blamed for being concerned that they be forced into social retirement long before they are ready. With women living one third of their years well beyond menopause, looking "old," which in our culture means doing without the cosmetics and clothes younger women are all too ready to use, is decidedly unrealistic.

Middle-aged and older women are no different from any other, and to the extent that they maintain contact with social situations, in addition to the habits established over the years, they must continue to pay attention to grooming and dress.

But being older carries with it both advantages and disadvantages. Experience over the years is likely to give more women than ever the sense of self and awareness of the nature of social encounters. The mature, stable woman, by the time she has reached her forties and fifties, has learned to distinguish between fashion and fad. She has a greater amount of experience with herself and how she would like to look, as well as with those things that make her feel most attractive and appropriately garbed. She knows which colors and cuts of clothes and hair style are most becoming both to herself and to her audience. Young girls, whether they can afford to or not, tend to experiment with numerous changes of clothes, cosmetics, hair styles, searching for an image of themselves they admire. The middle-aged woman is more likely to tell by a glance at the rack whether the particular cut, fabric, color of dress is for her. She has the advantage of being able to follow fashion at a distance, adopting the current to her particular style. She knows which looks get which responses: from men, from her women friends, from the people with whom she works.

Dressing for new roles can be a problem for middle-aged women as well if their earlier experience has been within a different milieu. The newly divorced suburban housewife, moving into the world of swinging singles might find she has to learn a whole new way of dressing; the woman moving into a career for the first time may find her old uniform of Bermuda shorts and roll-sleeve blouse no help at all; the woman whose struggling husband strikes it rich at mid-life may need much help in learning to dress for their new life style. For many of these women, "good taste" becomes an issue. Again, the mass media, the women's magazines, the manufacturers of cosmetics and clothes make it difficult for women to miss. And the range of goods they have provided comes in all sizes, prices, and shapes, making dress and grooming really far more *fun* for modern women than it ever was before—all of us now have available to us the potions and charms as well as costumes that in other times and places were only for princesses and queens and the very young, and forbidden or unavailable to others.

The budget beauty shops, the do-it-yourself coloring and blow-dry hairdos, the creams and lotions and pots of paints all beckon to women to stay with it—and they do help women of all ages look attractive. Even the less-than-well-endowed can use the skills of grooming and dress to compose an aesthetically satisfying picture. No longer is this artistry the province only of the very rich.

But, sadly, looking great at middle age may simply require more time and greater effort. This is not to say that young girls do not often spend an inordinately long time before the mirror and shopping as they learn the skills of assembling a desired appearance. But they can still manage to look great with a simple fresh look and few cosmetics. As she grows older, however, a woman begins to find she needs more cream to keep the skin smooth, some color to highlight the hair, and more grooming in general. On her the windswept look appears unkempt, the ungreased skin parched or wrinkled, the natural hair discolored, and the unpainted face dull. While there may be some nostalgic charm in the picture of Whistler's mother, hair tucked beneath her cap and in a rocking chair, middle-aged and older women of today hardly view this as the image of themselves. They know that such a picture represents retirement from life—no one will hire them or care to keep them on a job, regardless of the laws against discrimination. They know this is a look of resignation from the active world of work and sociability.

The cosmetic and clothing industries are indeed friends of middle-aged women. Younger women too are using, because of fashion, all the cosmetic tricks of the trade which older women find they must use to maintain their good looks. This generation of young girls is unlikely to forget grooming skills as they grow older; on the contrary, they will improve upon them. The middle-aged women of the future are likely to be more beautiful than ever as they maintain their active social lives, bringing to their social encounters the skills of dress and grooming developed over the years.

But not all is well, alas. The cosmetics industry can justifiably be accused of appealing to narcissism. But that is hardly the main quarrel with it. They can also be accused of making huge profits by creating overexaggerated needs. Their ads have appealed to some of the most exploitative of social relationships—images of well-kept sex kittens have abounded. The glamour magazines, catering to these advertisers, were, it is true, among the first to feature black girls epitomizing great beauty on their front covers and their pages, and well-dressed career girls helping overcome anti-"black is beautiful" attitudes and limited views of women's roles. But on the whole they portrayed a narrow view of the picture of the average woman. However, even these problems do not represent the worst difficulty with the cosmetics and fashion industries.

The greatest difficulty has to do with our health. Every woman who knows she must have swallowed hundreds of lipsticks in her life having made up before dinner cannot help but be angered by the knowledge that some of the dyes used in those lipsticks might be carcinogenic. And now we hear that some hair dyes are absorbed by the scalp, entering the blood stream, excreted by the bladder, and possibly carcinogenic.

Please, cosmeticians, we want to be your friends. Women are not apt to give up their paint pots and their hair colors. We like them too much, they are too useful to us. But keep them free of danger!

# A Social "Change of Life"

Every society in the world maintains some design concerning the way in which people of different ages in different stages of the life cycle are expected to behave in relationship with one another. These age structures vary from place to place, every cultural system creating its own pattern of movement from birth through maturity and eventual death, defining what it considers the appropriate behavior by styles of etiquette, by rights, and obligations. And every society tends to distinguish age sets by symbols; for example, dress. Ceremonials are often performed to mark transitions from one stage to another.

While modern society is remarkably more open in regard to what is considered acceptable behavior, even appropriate behavior—the choices open to us are far greater than ever before in the history of human society—still we cannot escape either the biological basis upon which this age differentiation is based or the particular knowledge and attitudes we have acquired in childhood and the traditions that have survived. We cannot escape the particular historical experience of our own generation, always somewhat different from the preceding generation and the generation to follow.

*Rites de Passage* are ceremonial ways by which traditional societies move persons from one stage of the life cycle to another. The life stages in these cultures are fairly strictly determined, and the ceremonies mark the transitions as people move from one stage to another. Each culture determines the significant stages to be marked—they may roughly approximate biological stages, but are not identical from place to place. A look at the traditional Hebraic stages illustrates the way in which these ceremonies serve as transition points. The young male child is first welcomed into the society via the ceremony of circumcision. At puberty he is welcomed into the congregation of adult males via the ceremony of Bar Mitzvah. The next major stage in his life is that of marriage. And at death, he is ceremonially removed from the world of the living by the prayers of Kaddish and the mourning ceremony of Shivvah.

In many societies all the boys born at approximately the same time are grouped in age grades; in some societies they undergo circumcision at puberty together with their age mates. Marriage is a ceremony practiced practically everywhere, as are ceremonies for death.

*Rites de Passage* are also practiced for women in many places. They may be for birth, first menstruation, first communion, marriage, motherhood, etc., the particular time and period of life so marked varying from place to place. But, curiously, there are no *Rites de Passage* for menopause! Yet there are plenty of indications that with menopause, women face not only a biological change but, in our society as well as in many others, changes in social status. These changes are marked by events similar to the *Rites de Passage*, and involve all the uncertainties and potential dangers involved in moving from one stage of life to another. We even have a phrase for this: "the change of life."

Anthropologist Van Gennep described these rites as they occurred in many societies.[1] He found that they were composed of three parts. The first involved separation from a previous status, the second involved a state of transition, often fraught with tension and danger, and the third involved incorporation into the new status toward which one was moved. This last stage, incorporation, usually involved being "claimed" by someone or something into that new station of life. A look at the traditional marriage ceremony illustrates these stages: the father "gives" the bride in marriage, she is removed thereby from his protection; and the groom "takes" the bride, claiming her for her new status as married woman and wife. In between, she is symbolically in a state of transition and, if stood up by the groom at the altar, is in considerable danger.

Society, in defining different life stages, also makes provisions for helping people over the hurdle from one stage to another. Even when people look forward to the next stage with anticipation and willingness, as for example young people might as they move to adulthood, there is generally trepidation and anxiety in the face of the unknown. The ceremonial *Rites de Passage* reflect the wisdom of mankind in devising ways of ritualizing the social support needed to enable us to forego the familiar former status and move on to the unfamiliar new.

More often than not people have little choice in the matter of moving through the life stages. For one thing, there does exist a biological base—the only alternative to the physical process moving us from birth through old age is premature death. For another, different age groups are capable of different functions. Among all mankind there exists the phenomenon of neotony—the prolonged real, physical dependency of the young we bear. Human infants need nurturance and assistance—their bodies as well as their mental abilities require a long period of development after birth before they are able either to physically reproduce, or intellectually maintain the necessary skills for survival of the society. The very old and senile are also generally incapable of performing the functions necessary to the survival of the group. For the people in between, each culture has devised some patterned system of duties and obligations for each group. Given the particular prestige or acclaim associated with that level, each group acts out the particular roles—acceptable behavior—associated with that status.

Also, by involving other social actors than ourselves, *Rites de Passage* serve to tell others how to behave toward us in our new position. Even if we feel no different, look little different, there comes a realization through the social behavior of others that now we are different.

The value placed on each age level varies from culture to culture. There does not seem to be any universal law that automatically proclaims youth superior in social position to age, or middle age superior or inferior to the healthy aged. And for women, the close of the reproductive period of their lives in no way automatically determines their declining status, prestige, and power in society. Indeed, in much of the world the reverse of the Western tradition holds true, the postmenopausal woman has more influence, freedom, and greater respect and prestige than ever.

There are few formal ritualized *Rites de Passage* in the traditional sense left in the secular world of industrial society. They have been replaced by secular symbolism that defines changing status; for example, a driver's license marks the younger adolescent off from the pre-adult youth, and marriage ceremonies are still with us although increasingly they are composed to suit individual tastes.

While there are no *Rites de Passage* in the formal, ritualized sense for women today, there is plenty of evidence that with middle age, women are made—by both physical signs and the actions of others—to recognize that they are moving over into a new status. And since that status in our society is *lower* than that of the younger women, for women to resist and resent these signs is hardly surprising. Even the most content, intelligent woman cannot help but notice that despite how well, attractive, good she feels, others let her know that her status is changing. Event after event is reinterpreted by others to enforce the new status.

No woman at middle age can help but notice these. When she mentions that a room is warm, there is bound to be someone who titters and makes a remark about hot flushes; should the twenty-year-old sitting in the next chair make the same remark about the warm room, the gentlemen are likely to rush to open the window or turn down the thermostat. And, indeed, the room might very well be hot. When a middle-aged woman is angry, nervous, irritable, others say *that* is menopause: that it might very well be an appropriate response to a real-life situation is too often a secondary consideration. If she exhibits signs of jealousy or is upset about the possibility her husband is having an affair, that is attributed to the paranoiac tendencies of menopause. I recall one woman in her late forties who, responding to what she felt a developing psychological distance between her husband and herself, one day burst into tears. He said, "You're so nervous. I think it's your menopause." That very afternoon, inadvertently answering the telephone from an extension, she overheard a conversation which proved her husband *was* having an affair.

The signs come from many directions. Often there is role reversal in relation to parents. Once they cared for you as a child; now you find yourself caring for them as the parent. There comes a time, also, when everyone else seems to look young—so different from the time when they all seemed older. Policemen begin to look like sons rather than fathers or older brothers. Shopping brings its public intimation of change of status—the male salespeople, young and older, take an inordinate amount of time with the young women customers and pay perfunctory attention to you. Men flirt with the daughter, not the mother. While young women are allowed their assortments of cosmetics and pills, your aches and pains become those of the cranky, menopausal lady. The extra attention needed with creams and other cosmetics are seen as weapons against the years rather than tools of the plastic art available to all. And keeping trim and firm and maintaining good skin and hair all seem to take more effort and

time. It's as if it is easier to spend the first half of your life developing your mind, the body seemingly effortlessly taking care of itself,
and the second half reversing the attention, needing now to take care
of the body.

Jokes about older women no longer seem so funny—after all that's
*you* they're laughing at.

And how one feels about oneself is only part of the picture, for
what really is happening is that all of these signs, and the social behavior of others toward one, are ways of pushing an age group out of
one status and off into another—one with little prestige in modern
Western society. The process takes time, and for women in the forties the picture may be less acute than for women in their fifties and
beyond. But it is part of the process of moving into the age group of
the old—a status with little power, prestige, and attraction in this society.

Novelist Doris Lessing described the way in which behavior of
others toward oneself reinforces this change of status. In her book,
*Summer Before the Dark*,[2] the heroine has been given a cat for a pet
by her family. Her husband was busy having his "fling." The children were grown and exerting their independence from "Mom." The
cat was ". . . just the thing for the menopause," they believed. And,
although the heroine was just forty and had not even begun to have
physical signs of menopause, ". . . it suited them to have me in that
stage," out of the way, no longer terribly important. The depressing
title of Doris Lessing's book, *Summer Before the Dark*, reflects an
unnecessary negative view toward mid-life. The implication of the
title is that of morbid anticipation. It reflects the notion that the period between middle age and death can be scarcely anything but a
period of decline, not only of physical but also of mental power; that
one moves from youth to old age through "the dark." Such an unfortunately negative approach to the menopausal years and the postmenopause can and does induce states of hypochondriacal depression. For many women, anxiety and anticipation can produce a
legion of complaints, many of which have no organic basis in the
biological facts of menopause but, rather, arise out of fear.

Recognition of the potential dangers of menopause as a social
state of transition is illustrated by the Spiritualist women of Swan-
sea, in England, who are noted for their seances and other efforts to
communicate with what they believe to be the spirit world. Member-

ship in these Spiritualist groups is largely female, and most of these women are middle-aged. According to one student of these Spiritualist meetings, a high proportion of the messages received from the "Spirit" could most obviously be interpreted as being related to menopausal symptoms.[3] But, interestingly enough, these were not symptoms associated with physical or medical problems. They dealt primarily with conditions of and feelings of uncertainty and lack of direction. Moreover, the Spiritualists explained, these so-called menopausal symptoms could occur at any time in a woman's life between the ages of twenty-four and onward. They were not associated merely with the end of childbearing ability or with the ending of menstruation. To the Spiritualists, menopause was seen as a cultural or social event rather than a biological truth. It could occur at any time a woman experienced a sense of change accompanied with uncertainty concerning the direction of her life. This sense of insecurity sent these women in search of answers from the "spirits" in an attempt to reach some understanding and accommodation with their roles in life. In effect they were defining menopause the same as "transition" or "passages," the period of movement from one status to another, the period in between, as noted by Van Gennep, fraught with danger.

With menopause, life is hardly about to end. But still many women in our society experience with intense awareness, especially as menopause approaches, the limited time ahead. Almost inevitably a reassessment of one's life is in order. The dreams unfulfilled, the things still undone, the clash between the reality of life and the desires for other things and ways, the children unborn, the lovers unloved, the talents undeveloped. For women, in the past, a reassessment of personality and life style was in many ways more difficult than for men. Women were more circumscribed than they are today in our society, learning to identify primarily with the home and childrearing. Dreams were repressed, creativity discouraged, and sublimation of desires to the needs of families considered appropriate. Still, for many, mid-life brought on a sense of "panic of the closing door,"[4] the sense that it was now or never, and with little opportunity to move beyond into the translation of dreams and fantasy into reality, hypochondria, depression, and other symptomology of intense dissatisfaction or fear were not surprising. For others, peaceful accommodation to the facts of life, an acceptance of prevailing con-

ditions, was more typical. Indeed for most, following the initial emotional distress and discomforts, the accommodation is expressed in
the serene quality typical of many old people.

But modern woman has *one third of her life to live* beyond actual
menopause! She is not about to sublimate, suppress, restrict the opportunity to live that period of her life joyously. Hypochondria and
depression are too wasteful of energies and hardly the stuff of
dreams. This eagerness to live fully and well has contributed to
women's impatience with physiology—an eagerness to grasp at medical panaceas to bring freedom from pain or discomfort.

As menopause approaches some women wish to have another
child, return to school, take a job, establish bonds with the world
outside in an effort to maintain participation—to retain contact with
life. It is at this time, in their forties, that many women experience a
renewed interest in sex, and engage in extramarital affairs, some to
assure themselves of continuing femininity, others because of released inhibitions and a desire to experience beyond the limitations
of their marriage.

All women are not the same, and all behavior does not have the
same causation. But more and more women, and men as well, living
in modern society and with increased life expectancy know that the
door is not closing, that life does go on, that thirty and forty years
stretch before one, and moving through the decades of the forties
and the fifties ought to be graceful, fulfilling, and need not necessarily be turbulent. With a little bit of luck, the health holds out
substantially well enough for continued sexual vigor, social participation, and self-realization. But these require self-confidence and
competence, and a refusal to accept a definition of oneself as useless.
A lifetime of training for flexibility, resiliency, is probably required.

There is little doubt, however, that with the approach of menopause, women, like men of similar age, are confronted with the need
to reassess who they are, where they are going, what they are doing
with their lives. There is the need to examine their values, the changing values of the world around them, and to make a reassessment of
where they stand and what they believe and how they wish to live
their remaining years. For some, the tasks are overwhelming. Loneliness, growing divorce rates at this age, exploitative sex relationships
in the world of the singles, economic insecurity, etc., are some of the
prices paid for plunging into the world beyond. For others, their en-

thusiasm, interest, and willingness to assume new risks and engage in
new ventures make their lives more exciting and fulfilling than ever.
And always there is the uncertainty that accompanies every transitional phase of life—leaving the known for the unknown—and never
quite sure if the world out there is ready to accept us on our new
terms.

Whether the emotional problems of some women at menopause
are the result of biological change or result from the social and psychological problems imposed by the society and the fact of our limited years on earth cannot yet be answered completely. There are
probably elements of all at work. For the physiologist there remains
the needed task of far more research than ever before. The laboratory of human experience, for the time being, has far more evidence
on its side, pointing to the varying positions of women in societies
throughout the world, and the critical nature of the mid-life period
as women move from one role to another, to higher or lower status.
That women respond to these shifts in their position is inevitable. As
women re-evaluate their lives and their values, "Who am I now and
for the future?" is the question increasingly asked.

Western industrial societies, along with many other peoples of the
world, have historically found the older woman expendable and paid
minimal attention either to her biology or her social needs. Other
peoples, in other places and times, have accorded positions of honor
and even power to women who have survived into later maturity.
There is nothing natural about the woman at menopause being either incompetent, unnecessary, unlovely, or unwanted and depressed.

It is clearly suspicious to consider "problems" of menopause as
universal, when there are plenty of societies in the world where
women do not see menopause as a problem—indeed, some don't
even have a word for it—and within our own society most women experience little or no difficulties whatsoever.

The question remains, why do some societies, including our own,
teach an anticipation of trouble and regard menopause as stigmatizing, whereas others do not? And how is it that most women have the
strength to resist such labelings?

One of the reasons offered for the lack of difficulty in some cultures is related to the changing status of women at this time of their
lives. In our own culture, growing older does not usually bring
greater social rewards. Among many other people in the world, on

the other hand, a picture quite opposite is the case. In many places it is only the older woman, past childbearing, who is permitted the respect and authority ordinarily only associated with men.

For example, among the Tuareg, the blue-painted people of the North African desert, the rituals of authority are not available to women. It is only when she grows older and is free of the responsibility of children, disassociated from childrearing and also from sexuality, that a woman can build up the respect that comes with authority. But what a price she is required to pay for the right to assume the authority and respect usually due men; she must, in effect, give up the symbol of her femininity—her sexuality and motherhood.

This is not so terribly different from the nineteenth-century customs concerning schoolteachers in much of rural America. A woman could hold the position—one of respect and some authority for the time—but only so long as she remained a spinster. Modern women are not about to accept that the roles of sexual being and mother are inevitably in conflict with those positions accorded high status in the society.

The Tuareg, incidentally, also maintain a custom to distinguish between the social classes and sexes. Since they are nomadic, all people have to travel together and isolation from the group is impractical. Anthropologist Robert Murphy points out that the veil—among the Tuareg worn only by the men—acts as a social barrier, covering their noses and mouths.[5] The higher status the man, the more strictly does he wear the veil. No lover is permitted to see his mouth. Dr. Murphy suggests that newspapers act in the same way to maintain social distance and separation between people; for example, in the subways during the rush hour, or at the breakfast table separating husband from wife, or when people spend time while kept waiting for a rendezvous or appointment.

In some ways, old women in our culture also have more freedom than the young to engage in certain behaviors, but not always because of greater respect. For example, an older woman can eat or drink alone in public places where a young woman's presence might appear to be an invitation.

Sociologist Pauline Bart has called the change in position in the society at mid-life, "Why Women's Status Changes in Middle Age, the Turns of the Social Ferris Wheel."[6]

Dr. Bart examined the data on some thirty societies around the world looking for those characteristics that indicated whether or not women's status changed at this time of their lives. More respect, special privileges, more freedom (especially from taboos), and more power and influence were considered to indicate higher status. Using these considerations, it was found that status went up in seventeen of the cultures, down in two, and didn't change in the remaining eleven. Why should these changes have occurred, and what were the factors influencing them? The answer lies largely in the roles women play at this time in their lives. A role refers to the rights and duties, the approved patterns of behavior for the occupants of a given position. Being a menopausal or postmenopausal woman implies different things in different cultures, for women of this age group do not necessarily have the same roles assigned to them universally. For example, to be in the position of a grandmother may be a biological fact, but the social role assigned to grandmothering may or may not exist. In some cultures grandmothers look after their grandchildren, in others they are occasional visitors or not even expected to maintain close relationships. Role adjustment experienced at this point of life can cause difficulty in some *but not all* societies, for some *but not all* women.

According to this analysis, most of the traditional role relationships of menopausal women in our society push us over into the category of those women who lose status in this period of their lives. Many of the factors that improve life for older women are either absent or not dependable.

Among the Pukapukans, the Navajo, and the Lovedu no menopausal difficulties are reported. In both the Navajo and the Lovedu women, a high position is maintained in the society throughout life; in all three, older people are looked to for leadership, and no stigma is attached to aging.

Those conditions of life leading to a raised status at menopause in the experience of other societies may seem somewhat surprising to us. They seem to point to characteristics different from our own culture, and include those things we are probably unable to accept for the future.

Among them is a strong tie of a woman with her own relatives as opposed to a system in which a marriage tie to a husband is stronger than a tie with one's family. Another is an extended family system as opposed to the smaller husband-wife nuclear family in which so much is invested in a relationship with very few people. Reproduction seems important as opposed to sex as an end in itself. This seems to be because a strong mother-child relationship, which is reciprocal in later life, insures a better life for older mothers than our own and other adult-oriented systems, which devalue strong attachments between children and parents. Institutionalized grandmother and mother-in-law roles are also associated with higher status for older women in contrast to the absence of those roles, or unimportance given them, again probably because of the built-in security and respect that come to older women as a result.

But if sex as an end in itself is not valuable for producing a family insurance plan, sex as an end in itself *after* menopause is *fun*, and to be encouraged. To value our sexuality without childbearing seems to point in the direction of higher status for women freed from the concern of possible pregnancy.

Sex as an end in itself before menopause seems to occur in those societies in which women's status goes down, as opposed to those places where reproduction is very important. The Trobriand Islanders of the South Pacific and the people of the Marquesas are in many ways similar to our own glamorous, sexually oriented culture where age is not valued. Young women were valued for their erotic skill and attractiveness. And a Marquesan girl, for example, like many of the sex kittens of our own time, could parlay her looks and sexiness into high positions within her husband's household—he could have more than one wife, but the sexiest could become the head wife. These women nursed their children as briefly as possible to keep their breasts beautiful, and babies were fed at the convenience of the adults—no demand schedules here. Old women did most of the women's work while the younger women entertained the men. And as far as menstruation was concerned, it not only did not interfere with sex, but one of the favored cures for prolonged menstrual bleeding was intercourse with the household head. Men didn't fare any better than women in this society, as far as age was concerned. A man was outranked by his son as soon as the child was born.

Living among one's own relatives appears to help in increasing status, again in contrast to a residence system that isolates women from their relatives and grown children. In general, of course, the valuing of age over youth heightens a woman's social position as she ages.

One of the more obvious factors that operates to devalue older women and which modern Western society shares, is the valuation of youth over age. Where age is valued over youth, growing older clearly has the advantage of increased respect and frequently increased power. Our youth-oriented culture, which during the decade of the 1960s had us "old" at thirty, doesn't help much in this regard. I recall one tongue-in-cheek movie that ended as the ten-year-olds were plotting to take the world away from the nineteen-year-old "elders." Fortunately, this is highly unlikely to happen, especially since the infants of the post-World War II baby boom period are now over thirty, and sooner than they may know that generation will be over forty and fifty. Their importance, simply in terms of the sheer pressure of their numbers, as a consumer market, which will turn the attention of the advertisers and commercial setters of style toward them, will make the middle years seem far more popular and important than ever before.

Bart did not find that economic roles seemed to be very much related to women's status. Women produce in every society, and unless their work is highly valued and given the same status as that of men, working by itself is no passage to high regard.

Modern life has moved in the direction of shifting women away from those roles which traditionally raised her status. Some women are caught in the midst of changing values, some gaining in strength, thrilling to the opportunity for growth and change; others collapsing under pressures for which they are unprepared.

Today's woman is in a sense a pioneer, for never before have so many been faced with the prospect of living out their lives without the traditional roles that charted the course of their aging. Women are not about to return to traditional systems, although they may find the independence of singlehood, childlessness, and physical autonomy more illusory than real as they grow older. At the same time, women are not about to fall apart at the prospect of carving new roles and life styles to suit an era of considerable prosperity, health, and choice. But that *some* women are likely to find the stresses involved in growing older without the traditional supports of family and homogeneous value systems overwhelming is not surprising.

A program of education to enable women to understand their bodies and the physiological significance of their menstruation and menopause will go a long way in alleviating many of the fears and apprehensions of women in this stage of life concerning the physical facts of life. But education alone will not change those social conditions that create in women apprehensions about their lives when they reach the middle years.

# The Many Roles of Women

Until recently, one of the very popularly believed reasons behind the cause of mid-life and menopausal difficulties was that women reached this period of their lives about the time that their children were grown and leaving home, the so-called "empty nest" syndrome. For women who had invested their lives, their time, emotions, and devotion to their children, no longer being needed was believed to have plunged them into the depths of despair.

There are many different kinds of women of all social classes and ethnic traditions. While an "empty nest" symbolized the end of the world for some, this was hardly the case for all. For a woman whose entire reason for living is her children, their departure from her—the loss of a sense of being needed on her part—with no preparation for other activities and skills can be traumatic.

The reality is that a large proportion of women in the United States by the time they reach menopause will have no children under the age of eighteen living with them. But the chances that these women's lives were so completely wrapped up in their children to the point that they experience mental breakdown as a result of the "empty nest" is hardly the major problem. More serious is the question of physical care and financial responsibility for aging parents in a society with fewer and fewer children in a family to share this frequent responsibility.

Slightly over one half of the women in the United States aged forty-five to fifty-four and over three fifths of the women aged fifty-five to sixty-four have had fewer than three children. Given modern life styles, which see most of the children off on their own and often in other parts of the country, it is clear that most women will experience an "empty nest." Many women, and their husbands, find this prospect rather delightful. Life without the children is not necessarily a life not worth living. And as our culture places more and more emphasis on the value of leisure, play, and romance, the chance for a couple to live together without the responsibilities of children in the household is scarcely a tragedy.

What is true is that a fairly substantial proportion of persons in the middle years have only a few, if any, offspring on which to call for supportive help, if needed, as old age and retirement approaches. And that aspect of an "empty nest" seems more significant than emotional ties to absent children.

Some women have always worked and had interests outside the home, and the numbers so involved in activities beyond the immediate confines of childrearing in this society are increasing over the last few generations. More than 42 per cent of all mothers in the United States hold jobs outside their homes. According to the U. S. Labor Department, while the number of *working women* has doubled since just before World War II, the number of *working mothers* has increased eight times! The occupations of working mothers are similar to those of all women in the work force. Of every one hundred working mothers, there are thirty-two clerical workers, twenty-two service workers, fifteen factory operatives, sixteen professional workers, eight sales workers, and seven in other occupations.

The 1970 census reports that women accounted for two thirds of the increase in total employment in the 1960s, and for half or more of the gain in certain jobs, ranging from bookkeeping to bartending. There has been a shift from the more servile occupations to those with higher status. For example, the number of women reported working as maids dropped more than one-half million during the decade, while the number of women working in clerical jobs rose 3.8 million.[1]

The experiences of women with a world larger than the immediate confines of children and the household extend to interests and even power once considered primarily male enclaves. For example, in 1975 the New York Stock Exchange, one of the major financial trading institutions in the world, announced that the typical shareholder is a fifty-three-year-old woman who lives in a large metropolitan area such as Chicago or New York. According to the report, she is a member of a household with a combined income of $19,000 a year, holds a professional or technical job, has spent four or more years in college, and has a portfolio worth $10,500. Still, with 40 per cent of the jobs in America held by women, the vast majority are relatively low level. And women's incomes lag an average of $3,500 a year below that of men.

Despite their legal rights to participate, women still play a relatively minor role in the active political life of the nation. In a 1976 study of women officeholders done at the Center for the American Woman and Politics at Rutgers University, New Jersey, it was pointed out that women hold fewer than 5 per cent of the elected offices in the nation. Even in those offices usually thought of as being appropriate to women, such as school board membership, women hold a tiny minority of positions. Only 13 per cent of elected school boards were women; 4 per cent of the members of state senates, and 9 per cent of the lower houses of state legislatures are women.[2] But there is now a momentum established by the post-World War II generation; with increasing numbers of women entering occupations outside the home, including the more prestigious occupations, the chances that their numbers will continue to increase remain high.

The numbers of women entering the work force are influenced by such factors as rising divorce rates, the climate of acceptance of women's right to work outside the home, lowered esteem for the traditional housewife role, and Federal laws concerning equality of hiring opportunities.

Most women, as throughout history, work because they participate actively in the common task of earning a livelihood and maintaining a desired standard of living. More and more older women seek to enter the work force as they are confronted both with the need to help support themselves and their families. Also, they search for ways to continue active participation in social and economic life in the world outside the home itself. While large numbers of older women seek to enter the work force as their families mature, many women have always worked. Women accustomed to participating in the work force seem to maintain this involvement as long as they can. And women whose educational achievements and level of skill are high tend to stay in the work force both because they find this way of life in keeping with their view of themselves, and because high earnings are conducive to continuing employment.

These working women comprise all adult ages of course. But the lesson for the future seems clear. More and more modern American women will, by the time they reach middle age and menopause, have experience with far more than the one role of being a mother. They will have been workers, employers, have dealings with persons outside the home, have had experience earning their livelihood, contributing to the support of their families, and testing their abilities among others in the world outside. While their choices and options may be limited by their age, education, ethnicity, race, intelligence, skills, as well as social prejudice, this still is not the picture of the woman plunged into a state of nothingness as her children grow and leave home. And it would seem that, while depression will not be absent for some women, under the most ideal of conditions, the fact remains that among modern women the "empty nest" syndrome is likely to be more and more of an anachronism.

Curiously, most of the common status and role definitions described for women, in most societies, are a function of either their age or their relationship to men, such as their husbands and sons. One point of view to explain this is the women are "conceived almost exclusively as sisters, wives and mothers. Whereas men achieve rank as a result of explicit achievement, differences among women are generally seen as the product of idiosyncratic characteristics, such as temperament, personality and appearance,"[3] and it tends to neglect the real contributions made by women in the life of the group outside of their familial roles.

This is hardly because women have been unimportant in other areas. On the contrary, throughout time women have participated in economic production, helping the group to survive, as well as men. In almost all societies, including those based on hunting—an occupation almost exclusively male—women have provided an average of over 40 per cent of the food supply![4] And in contemporary American society, over 50 per cent of the women are in jobs outside the home.

The neglect of this view of women as workers, producers, and significant participants in the world outside the home is in part attributable to the myopic view of societies as they were observed from the view of the male-dominated European society, and the limited experience of women's roles in recent Western history.

Still, the association of women primarily in kinship relationships continues—it is the mother, wife, sister, etc., who is extolled, rather than the shopkeeper, seamstress, professor, or lawyer who happens also to be mother, wife, etc. There is no question but that woman's familial roles continue to affect our lives deeply as we live through the modern period of extraordinary changes in value systems and roles played.

## Motherhood

Despite the fact that in modern society children are expected to leave home and be on their own once they have reached adulthood, motherhood and mothering is one role that never seems to end. The "empty nest" syndrome may no longer be true because mothering, in and of itself, may no longer be the prime role in the life of a woman, especially by the time she has reached the middle years. Still, attachments to and responsibilities for children go on and on.

Modern women often experience serious conflicts in their mother role. They are wives too. Husbands frequently, especially at middle age, begin to make demands on their wives for increased attention and affection, and view the wife's involvement with teen-aged children or young adults still around the house as an intrusion, as competitive to their own needs, peace, and comfort. Mothers are often caught in the interplay of culture change—their own mothers watching and moralizing, the children moving in strange and new directions. Frequently, mothers are cast in the role of mediators between the generations, forced to defend or excuse their children's behaviors to grandparents, sometimes finding the grandparents defending and excusing the children to the detriment of the mother's control over their conduct.

Then there is the generation of mothers caught between the feminist trends of the 1920s and the liberated woman's movement of the 1960s; having themselves devoted the major part of their adult lives to the care of children and home. What a slap in the face to these women from those children who now put down mothering, who ask, "What else did you do?"

This is not the first generation of mothers in the world to experience the pangs and despair or joys and exhilaration often involved as society and culture change. The experience of post-World War II mothers is not unlike those generations everywhere caught between the passing of one set of traditions and the development of the new.

And the mothering responsibilities go on and on. With increasing rates of divorce, adult children often return. More significantly, they turn their children over to mother, now grandmother. There is an old folk saying, "Little children, little problems; big children, big problems." Mothers can abandon children at any time of course, but for almost all of us, mothering goes on forever.

## Mothers and Sons

Perhaps no other close relationship is as stigmatized in modern Western society as the relationship between a mother and son. Sigmund Freud didn't help the image of an intimate mother-son relationship very much when he termed the "Oedipus Complex," often used to describe the love and attachment of an adult male child to his mother, implying an instinctive urge toward incest in this relationship. The ancient Greek King Oedipus has been much maligned in this regard—after all he didn't *know* he was marrying his mother. Philip Wylie, writing after World War II, also attacked "momism," impugning evil and castrating motives to adoring and affectionate mothers. And the poor Jewish mother has been the butt of jokes, an object of scorn held for all to deride in novel after novel, on film and in the cabaret.

How curious are the ways of mankind. Ours is a culture which tells mothers: "Release your children, let them be on their own, build your lives around relationships with those outside the family and activities not dependent on kinsmen." For those who, whether because of tradition, affection, or simply need, find it difficult to do so, we have little in the way of either sympathy or understanding, but rather respond with sneers and labels—neurotic, domineering, bossy, castrating, etc.

But mother-son relationships cannot be understood simply as neurotic, or affectional attachments. They primarily represent social attachments, defined and elaborated in different ways in different cultures and at different times. The experiences which middle-aged women have in relation to their sons and society's attitudes can be seen, from a cultural perspective, to have many different possibilities and ramifications.

The negative attitudes toward mother-son relationships in our society really reflect an effort to reinforce the breakdown of the extended kinship group and to support the nuclear family, consisting of husband, wife, children. A grown son, ideally in this culture, is expected to be off on his own or married with children of his own, with primary responsibility and affection for *his* wife and children. Attachment to his mother is considered adequately expressed by flowers or a telephone call on Mother's Day, a conveniently institutionalized occasion for remembering that there is a woman around who did bring him to life. Hopefully, *that* woman should not need him for company, medical care, financial assistance, emotional support, friendship, etc.

This kind of ideally distant relationship, of course, is not always the case in fact—else why all the complaining about mothers or about sons. Nor is it necessarily the case for all women in all societies and times.

For women who have little power or positions of their own, especially in those societies when at marriage they go off to live in their husband's households, often it is only when sons are grown and important, and their mothers by then middle-aged, that the women feel a measure of security and higher status. For example, among the Greek Sarakatsani—shepherds living in the mountains of northern Greece and southern Yugoslavia—women's status does not improve markedly until her sons are grown and married, and her own well-being at middle age is very much dependent on that fact.[5] As young girls the women are taught to limit their movements, walk modestly, never run, and be confined to the home. Eye contact with men is carefully avoided as it is thought to signify an invitation to sexual assault. Upon marriage she enters a hostile and distant household, that of her husband's family. Even close relations between husband and wife, which might relieve her loneliness, are resented by the other villagers—insistent that the husband's prime attachments be to his kinsmen and fellows rather than his wife.

For the Sarakatsani woman the major joy in life is the son who grows up. It is he who will support her, guaranteeing her comfort in old age. When her sons marry, they take over their father's position as head of the household, and for the first time since her marriage, a Sarakatsani woman's power and privileges are heightened, while those of her husband wane. Since her total relationship to the husband was one of subservience, with inability to complain for fear of hurting her son's future, she cannot help but invest her life in her son. How useless would be the admonitions of the Philip Wylies and Sigmund Freuds to these women. They know where their bread is buttered.

The increased status that women achieve as a result of having sons —particularly when their sons marry—is found in many societies around the world. Among the Coniagui of Africa, the women sing a joyful song when their sons marry and bring wives home to live—this too is a society where a bride goes off to live with her husband and his family. The song goes, "I shall no longer go to fetch wood and to fetch water; I shall no longer pound the grain." Here a woman sets greater store by her children, who will retain primary attachment to her rather than to her husband, whose primary attachment is to his own blood relatives and his own mother.[6]

This stands in contrast to our own society in which we consider that a man's first attachment is to his wife, and we therefore read something nasty or sick into a man's attachment to his mother. I recall a conversation about a man, himself middle-aged, who made an expected daily telephone call to his mother. One of the persons hearing that said, "Imagine, a grown man calling his mother daily. What a demanding mother." The reaction was one of derision of both the woman and her son. Yet the mother, over eighty years of age, living alone in the anonymous environs of a large city tenement, clearly needed someone to check on her well-being as well as to give notice of interest in whether or not she was alive. Still, our society teaches us that these attachments should not exist, when in point of fact they do.

Attachments between mothers and sons are not criticized only in our own society. Among the traditional peoples of Algeria, sons, after marriage, live with their father under the same roof, frequently three or four generations of an *ayla* or family living together. There may be as many as fifty people enclosed from the outside world living under conditions of intimacy and strict modesty. A mother can eat only with her son, no other male. Modesty prevents the mention of the names of wives among kinsmen, and the veil is worn by women; they are described as "like animals, highly sexed and willing to have intercourse with any man. That is all they care about." Thus, the only man with whom she is permitted close attachment is her son, no other male. Yet, women are considered troublemakers who will favor their own sons over the *ayla* and over the children of their husbands' other wives. Therefore, a woman must be guarded against. There is an Algerian proverb: "The Angel and the Man work for unity; Satan and the Woman for division." It is no wonder that a woman is pleased when her sons marry; now she holds authority over her daughters-in-law. At menopause these women are released from the pressures and restraints of their seclusion. They can wander outside the enclosed household, and have the independence denied them during their period of childbearing.[7]

Perhaps no mother in all of history has had more abuse heaped upon her than the Jewish mother. And you don't even have to be Jewish to fall into the stereotype picture of what such a woman is supposed to be like—domineering, castrating, overambitious, pushy, attempting to live her life through her children and, at the same time, ready to battle the world in praise and defense of her children over all others.

There is an old joke, with many variations, that describes the devotion of these women to their children.

Two Jewish mothers met in the supermarket and one asked the other how her children were doing. The other answered, "My daughter is married to such a wonderful man. He brings home good money. He shops and cooks and takes care of the children. She lives like a queen. My son, he's married to such a lazy good-for-nothing. All day he works so hard to make a living. When he comes home he has to shop and make supper and take care of the children."

While traditional Jewish women had strong attachments to their daughters, generally in the expectation that they will be companions and helpmates over the years, their great joy was in the accomplishment of their sons. Zborowski and Herzog, describing the Jewish ghetto communities of Eastern Europe in their popular book *Life is with People*, point to some of the traditional roots of the mother-son relationship.[8] In these communities the women held an extraordinary amount of influence. They were strong, self-confident mothers, and sons were their loyal supporters. The women controlled the family pocketbooks, directing the family spending. In the wealthier families women frequently worked, usually as shopkeepers, their husbands and sons frequently free to engage in scholarly pursuits. The women's greatest joy was to bear male children, and for those children to become scholars was deeply desired. Scholars were not necessarily influential people, but they epitomized the cultural ideal of a life of learning, and were a source of pride and moral value to their mothers. Mothers encouraged their sons toward excellence in their endeavors.

Several years ago the actress Shelley Winters portrayed a stereotyped American-Jewish mother, unwilling to let go of her son, prying and overseeing every aspect of his life, in the film *Next Stop Green-*

*wich Village.* In the film the mother eventually, but reluctantly and tearfully, bid her aspiring actor son good-bye with the admonition, "Be a *good* actor." What might have been a sensitive, sympathetic portrayal of a conflict of cultural attitudes between mother and son was somewhat spoiled by the overdrawn, cartoonlike joke of the Jewish mother.

Shelley Winters, in real life, knows differently. On a television talk show some years ago, after listening to conversation about the negative qualities of the "Jewish" mother, as portrayed in books like *Portnoy's Complaint,* etc., in exasperation she exclaimed: "What's so wrong with Jewish mothers? They make their sons doctors, lawyers, teachers. What's so terrible about that!"

Our society does not particularly value the continuity between generations and the persistence of tradition. The fragile nature of family relationships encourages the disparagement of deep ties between relatives, especially between mothers and sons. Sons are supposed to be socialized into the male world of the larger society outside the family. Mothers, especially mothers out of traditional ethnic, non-urban, non-industrialized, non-highly educated backgrounds are not considered capable of doing that. And even where they are, by virtue of their intelligence, education, and wisdom, suspicion of warmth between mother and son pervades the thinking of many. Mothers and grown sons can love each other and be good friends. To make a nasty joke out of a complex set of social factors influencing their relationship is indeed sad.

## Mothers and Sons-in-law

While the relationship between a mother and son has often been associated with deep emotion and open to interpretations of neurotic involvement, the relationship between a woman and her son-in-law has been one big funny joke. No comedian in the Western world, and many other places as well, is without his repertoire of mother-in-law jokes; no topic is as sure to get as loud guffaws except perhaps menopause itself.

Now, many women know they get along perfectly well with their sons-in-law, especially when they maintain a polite distance between one another. But why is the wife's mother so vulnerable to this role, forced to be the butt of humor and suspicion of questionable motives in her behavior even where she bears no ill will whatsoever to her daughter's husband? Why is the easiest and safest relationship one that involves a measure of non-involvement between the middle-aged woman and her daughter's husband?

Basically, it could be argued that a joke or avoidance are safer than open hostility. The mother-in-law/son-in-law relationship can carry within it the seeds of antagonism. Fun or distance are ways to dissipate the anger and possibility of open conflict between these actors playing roles in this social relationship.

Under the conditions of modern life, when a young couple go off to live on their own, establishing their own households, there may seem to be little reason for any possible conflict between sons-in-law and mothers-in-law. But we do bear in our thinking and in our behavior carry-overs from earlier traditions and periods in which mother-in-law avoidance or joking relationships were common. And even today we often hear a young man saying to his bride, "I married you, not your mother," or "I married you, not your relatives." (But we *do* marry our relatives in part.) A contractual marriage relationship carries with it the conditions of almost any social or business contract—specific rights and duties are outlined, specific obligations are assumed. A true contractual relationship in the words of the great anthropologist Radcliffe-Brown, in his analysis of joking relationships and avoidance relationships, is one in which ". . . the two parties are conjoined by a definite common interest in reference to which each of them accepts specific obligations."[9] Thus, at marriage a man and his wife assume obligations toward each other.

There are times, however, when the social structure is organized in such a way that a mother-daughter relationship can impose obligations on a daughter which can interfere with her obligations to her husband. The interests of mother-in-law and son-in-law are thus often contradictory and can lead to conflict or hostility. A mother may demand time, affection, friendship, even money, medical attention, etc.; a husband can be demanding the same or similar things of his wife—the mother's daughter. The mother can impose standards of behavior, influence over children, household affairs, or even the son-in-law's affairs, while he may be wishing to impose these standards on his own. Innumerable women have experienced the tugs and pains of maneuvering between loyalty to mother and loyalty to husband or loyalty to her side of the family—the relatives with whom she grew up and to whom she may have attachments as opposed to his side of the family—a family of strangers. The husband, demanding that loyalty be his, responds either by simply avoiding his mother-in-law or joking with or about her.

Paradoxically, avoidance and joking are ways of keeping things "cool," of maintaining friendship with mother-in-law rather than allowing matters to deteriorate into open hostility or conflict, which might even result in the breakup of his own marriage.

Among the native peoples of Australia, avoidance of mothers-in-law is carried to an extreme—a man carefully avoids *all* social contacts with his wife's mother. In that regard he is not necessarily different from many natives of Chicago or Los Angeles. But in Australia the men are careful also to express their great friendship for the mother of a wife. Indeed, mother-in-law is called "my greatest friend" because, after all, "she gave me my wife."

Modern women recognize the familiarity of the Australian pattern of avoiding contact in order to maintain friendship. Friendship, after all, represents the obligation *not* to enter into open quarrel or conflict. For some people the only way to get along is simply to avoid each other by mutual agreement. Among the Australians and many other people, this is a socially defined, required behavior, enabling a woman's mother to stay on good terms with her daughter's husband.

Joking is somewhat different from avoidance. Anyone who has ever heard a mother-in-law joke, and heard the titters in the audience, cannot help but be aware that joking is a form of sham conflict —a way of fighting without having to engage in real conflict. The mother-in-law often represents the enemy because her daughter's relationship to her may stand in conflict with the daughter's obligations to the husband.

There is also the matter of sex. Despite all the social strictures against the older woman-younger man relationship, we know perfectly well that there is nothing natural about this. It is quite possible for a wife's mother to find her son-in-law a desirable sexual partner. He might even find her more attractive and interesting than his younger wife. Avoidance, sham hostility, all reinforce the taboos against the sexual involvement between a man and his wife's mother.

Modern men and women may make a real effort to extricate themselves from the traditional taboos and attitudes regarding mothers-in-law. But traditions die hard, and the conditions of modern life have not removed all the conditions that might lead to conflict of interests between these two partners in the social game. "I married you, not your mother" simply doesn't hold true when mother requires financial, emotional, or other assistance. A mother-in-law may be widowed or divorced, and with the smaller number of children in the modern nuclear family, her daughter may be the relative she depends on for many things. Involvement with her daughter's family is a way of fending off loneliness. One's children do have a grandmother—and mother-in-law once more enters the picture in regard to family life. And there is always the real possibility that the emotional ties between daughter and mother may supersede in strength the ties between wife and husband.

Middle-aged, menopausal women, as mothers-in-law may very well be quite innocent in all this drama. They may be happy for their daughters in relation to their marriage partners; they may be nondemanding financially, emotionally, or socially. They may be the greatest. The chances remain, however, that the society around them will be unwilling to give up the attitudes, the bad jokes, the strained relationships. Middle-aged woman as mother-in-law finds her role laid out for her. It takes real understanding and patience to sort out the rights and obligations owed by a daughter-mother team from those owed the husband-wife team. Our society stresses that husbands come first. This is not always easy for women whose mothers really need them. The mothers themselves are caught in this social system. It looks as if the best way to get along with sons-in-law is not to take too much offense at the jokes—better that than real conflict. And it helps to remember that at times polite distance is the best way to maintain friendship. Better the occasional dinner and event shared together than the ultimate practiced by the Australian natives —open avoidance.

## Mothers and Daughters

There is an old proverb that goes, "My son's a son till he gets him a wife, my daughter's a daughter all of her life."

This seems to apply more readily, however, to situations where daughters do not leave to live with their husband's families (patrilocal residence) but rather stay close to mother. Yet, even in many societies where daughters leave, mother and daughter tend to come together at important times like childbirth—even today flying across a continent to be with daughter when she has her baby. Emotional ties between mothers and daughters often remain very strong.

Michael Young and Peter Willmott, in an excellent study of family and kinship in East London during the late 1950s, have described the very close bonds that exist between mothers and their married daughters.[10] Among these working-class residents of East London, the marriage of a daughter did not precipitate the "empty nest" syndrome described elsewhere, for the tendency was for the newly married couple to live with or near the wife's mother. For one thing, the husband's mother was considered to be too difficult to live with for she was a relative stranger to the woman and thus had unfamiliar housekeeping methods. The preference on the part of the couple was to live near the wife's parents, not with them, although a daughter who had married late, when the mother had no or fewer children left at home, might join the parental household.

In any event, married daughters and their mothers spend a good deal of time with each other, shopping together, having afternoon tea together, visiting one another, and sharing meals.

Devotion to "Mum" was understood as a normal, natural thing. "Mum" held the family together—after her death brothers and sisters were less likely to be close to one another. "Mum" helped when her daughter gave birth, she helped in child care, and took over the major responsibility for the household tasks when others in the family were at work.

The old proverb, "My son's a son till he gets him a wife, my daughter's a daughter all of her life," seems an appropriate description for the lives of these Londoners. Yet, under certain conditions, a young couple might turn to the husband's mother, rather than the wife's. In one case, for example, a young woman was impressed with the unsuitability of her mother playing the role of mother to married daughter, for the mother had a young child similar in age to a child of the couple's. In another, a daughter felt her mother played favorite to a sister. And there were cases where the husband's mother was widowed and was able to play the role of "Mum" better than the girl's mother, who had many children.

On the whole, these London women, when they reached their forties and fifties, if they had had daughters, which they were likely to have had since their family size was large, were assured of companionship and a continuing participation in the lives of succeeding generations. One did not lose a daughter, one gained a son.

What about the girl's husband and his relationship to wife's "Mum"? The relationship can indeed be somewhat tense. Husbands sometimes resent their wives' attachment to "Mum," and the amount of time spent with her. But open hostility is rare, and there is a tendency for men to be drawn into their wives' families. The possibility for conflict is, nevertheless, present. And as the structural anthropologist Radcliffe-Brown has pointed out, this situation requires some degree of limitation, control, and resolution. For those men who do not care to become closely enmeshed in their wives' families, some degree of mother-in-law avoidance is practiced. For the young couple, competition for loyalty by the husband and "Mum" for the loyalties of the daughter-wife can create a good deal of storminess in a marriage.

Even greater threats to the mother-daughter relationship has appeared from sources other than the daughter's husband. As people move upward in social class and education, there is a decreasing community of interest—better educated daughters are likely to be more interested in work and outside activities than time spent socializing with mother. There is a tendency for single grown daughters, as well as married daughters, to move away from the parents' home —to the suburbs or other cities, sometimes across continents. While the telephone replaces "dropping in," physical distance does have effects.

With children grown, some mothers now wish to invest their time and energies in their own education, careers, hobbies, friends, husbands, or new romances. Daughters who remain—who continue to require their mother's full attentions—can interfere with these pursuits.

All women are not the same. Today's middle-aged mother may wish her daughters to depend on her; others are pleased at their independence. One mother may be supportive of her daughter's new life styles, while another sees them as tragic breaks with tradition.

Modern mothers are so often struck by the liberated life open to their daughters but not experienced by themselves. Sometimes the mother enjoys her freedom vicariously. One such mother said of her daughter, "I hope she doesn't marry too soon. I'd like for her to *live*, to experience first." Her husband responded, "What do you mean, 'live'—to sleep with ten men instead of one?"

This mother may have meant that, but more likely she meant for her daughter to postpone marriage in favor of increased preparation for greater options in her life. But this is a mixed blessing. There are real fears and worries parents feel for the unmarried—especially the unmarried daughter. This is not so much any longer out of concern for the horrors of being an "old maid." Rather, it is the real wish for someone to love, care for, be responsible for the daughter—a mixture of desire for her safety and happiness, and a wish to be relieved of anxiety. The old order is gone; careers and freedom of movement carry with them continued responsibility by the parents for monitoring the well-being of the child. Friends and strangers assume some of this caring, but when the chips are down, it is people in the family who remain most committed.

The modern mother faces the difficult task of balancing her sentimental attachments to daughters and responsibility for them, with awareness that today's young women need to develop capacities and resources for independent lives. The mother must deal not only with the daughter's new life style, but with her own needs and desires at this time of her life.

## Mothers and Daughters-in-law

Relationships between a middle-aged woman and her son's wife, like so many other familial associations, are in the modern world usually characterized by polite distance. After all, in the monogamous, nuclear family, mother-son attachments are competitive with husband-wife attachments. While both women share affection and concern for the son/husband, inevitably some distance is likely to be demanded by the daughter-in-law in order to establish her priority in these matters.

This has not always been the case nor is it the same everywhere. And indeed, the rising divorce rate with the tendency for children to go with their mothers requires that grandmother/mother-in-law have friendly relations with daughter-in-law if she wishes continued social and affectional ties with the grandchildren.

Mother-daughter-in-law relationships in much of the world have something of the evil stepmother-poor Cinderella quality about them. This has generally been true in some, though not all, of the places where women had to leave their own blood relatives and mother to go off to live in the strange households of their husbands. This, combined with male dominance, strict authority, and even cruelty, and a low status during the early years of marriage, seems to invoke in these women a desire to impose their will and authority when their sons marry and bring home their wives. Moving from daughter-in-law to mother-in-law provides relief from drudgery as well as the psychological relief of now being the dominant rather than the subordinate person among the women in the household.

The old Chinese family was a classic example of this kind of relationship. The cruel mother-in-law played in Chinese fiction and folklore the role that the wicked stepmother played in European fairy tales. Among the traditional Chinese it was not unusual for the parents to arrange the marriages. If it turned out that they didn't like the girl once she came to live in the household, they could break up the marriage.

> A marriage is made in the name of the parents taking a daughter-in-law, not in the name of the son taking a wife. There is to be no expression of erotic life between any couple. . . . If there is a quarrel between his parents and his wife, a man has no alternative but to take the side of the older people against his wife. A woman's first duties are to her husband's parents; only secondarily is she responsible for her husband. She is expected to submit to her husband as she submits to her parents-in-law and her father.[11]

The domination of the mother-in-law over the girl was reinforced by the Confucian doctrine of respect for age which is written in the *Li Chi*, the *Book of Ritual*.

While evil mothers-in-law represent the ogre figure to girls forced to leave their families for life within the authoritative structure of a strange household, for a mother to be involved in arranging the marriage of her son can also serve to insure that the women sharing the household be compatible one with the other. Not all Chinese mothers-in-law were mean, of course. It is true, however, that conditions in the Chinese family lent themselves to this as a real possibility. Younger women were more open to exploitative behavior in the family than the older, who could now dominate others.

Among the Kurds, a Moslem people of Kurdistan, a woman helps arrange the marriage of her sons, and no bride would be chosen without her approval.[12] In the case of the Kurds, unlike the traditional Chinese, however, this power of a woman to choose her daughter-in-law facilitates strong female solidarity within the family. The girls chosen by the mother-in-law join the female household, which among the Kurds is largely secluded from the males, doing their household work in fellowship and enjoying their social life together. A song proudly sung by the women says: "Many families have wanted us, many men we say have wanted us." These women do not present a picture of disgruntled, cranky women waiting for their chance to get even by exploiting younger women. The Kurdish society practices careful segregation of the sexes, the men leading a life including the outside world, the women confined to the household. Men can come and go to the cafes, the streets, the park; women traveling out no more frequently than once a week. The women provided their own amusements at home, daughters-in-law included.

Great respect for her in-laws is also expected of the Toda woman of India, a society in which traditionally one woman married a group of brothers, in the custom known as fraternal polyandry. At the funeral of a young Toda woman, in the chanting of all the sins she could possibly have committed, two especially designated were "sleeping on a bed and letting one's father-in-law sleep on the ground" and "sitting on the veranda and driving one's mother-in-law from it."[13]

Among the Hopi and Navajo Indians of the American Southwest, a very different kind of relationship existed between mothers-in-law and their sons' wives. In both of these societies, descent and inheritance was through the female line, from mother to daughter. In addition, when a son married he went off to live in his wife's mother's household or camp. The children of the marriage were considered members of the mother's family group, rather than that of the father. Thus, a woman was likely to have a son-in-law around rather than a daughter-in-law. Mother-daughter-in-law relationships were therefore distant. When a son's marriage entered some difficulty he could always come home to mother and his own kinsmen. Daughters stayed home even after marriage.

In our own society women may have difficulties with their daughters, but there is, nonetheless, greater familiarity and emotional pulls and tugs than there is in the mother-in-law-daughter-in-law relationship. To interfere with a daughter-in-law's household routines—

to check on the housekeeping, look in the closets, comment on the rearing of children—is clearly looking for trouble. A woman is forced to be on greater guard in this relationship.

The relationship is complicated when there are grandchildren involved.

## Grandmother Role

For many of the women of the world, to become a grandmother is to have reached the high point of life. Among the women of Burundi in Africa, for example, a woman and her son-in-law address each other as "noble" once she has arrived at this station.

To be a grandmother brings with it, ordinarily, a sense of great achievement. One's children have grown, taken their positions in the adult world, and produced the generation that gives one the sense of continuing society, of continuing life.

And grandchildren can be fun. They can be joked with, played with, instructed with the wisdom of experience—and usually can be returned to parents for full-time responsibility.

But grandchildren-grandparent relations have never been completely without their complications. And with the nuclear family, plus the increasing rates of divorce among married couples with young children, problems for modern grandparents are increasing.

Grandparents take on many different roles in different cultures around the world. Some of these are familiar to us in our own society, others are not and their appearance among ourselves sometimes causes problems. Some of these relationships include joking or teasing; sometimes grandparents are expected to adopt or fully care for a child over a period of years; grandparents are often expected to socialize the child—to instruct him in the ways of the culture; in others grandparents are responsible for overall general care; and frequently an indulgent relationship is encouraged.

In her examination of the status of menopausal and post-menopausal women in thirty different societies, Pauline Bart found that in only two of these cultures the status of women decreased after menopause, and it was in these two societies that there were no close grandparent-grandchild relationships. In one of these, among the people of the Trobriand Islands, the fathers took care of the children—grandmother was superfluous. Among the Marquesans of the South Pacific, also, daughter's husband took care of the children and, again, grandmother was not needed to fulfill this function.[14]

There may very well be a lesson in this for our society. Our emphasis is on a two-generation, nuclear family. We emphasize mother, father, and children, plus companionship between husband and wife and their co-operation in childrearing. Grandmother has thus become less necessary and her role has become amorphous. Her efforts to raise the grandchildren are often interpreted as "meddling," her affectionate indulgent relationship with grandchildren called "spoiling," her lessons "old-fashioned." Many a middle-aged woman, having become a grandparent, is shocked and hurt by this relegation to the visit by appointment, and the message "don't get too close."

For other women, the picture is somewhat different. Glad to see their children grown and off, divorce catapults grandmother back to what our society considers the mothering responsibility, full-time care of the grandchildren. For some women this represents a real intrusion into the new companionate relationships between their husbands and themselves—once again child care supersedes the lover-companion-friend relationship. Two o'clock feedings, thought a thing of the past, come as an unwelcome surprise in middle age. For some women this brings on an enormous sense of guilt, as if they somehow had mismanaged the raising of their own children only to be punished by the failure of those children's marriages. Sometimes it brings on embarrassment. How do you, at age fifty-two, explain to friends that you can't go out with them because the sitter didn't show?

Many women are now finding that grandparenting is becoming an unexpected, sometimes unwelcome, extension of the mothering role. It is one thing to have raised your own children, given of time and energy and finances, finally to see them off into families of their own as is the ideal in our society. To visit the grandchildren occasionally, to baby sit but be able to return the babies to their mothers, to have weekend visitors but to be free the rest of the week, to feed and nurse on occasion but not as a full-time vocation as was the case with one's own children, are all parts of the pleasures. But when divorced, working mothers turn their children over to grandma full time, or when the divorced son's wife goes off with the children separating them from grandparents, the pleasures can turn to grief. And, with conflicts over how grandchildren should be raised "properly"—a frequent bone of contention between grand-parents and parent, especially in this world of rapidly changing values—grandmother often finds that her position is not one of respect and high status, as it has been traditionally in many cultures of the world, but is devalued and demeaned.

There are many groups of people within this society for whom grandparenting remains a significant, highly respected role. Among some American black families, it is the three- and sometimes four-generation family—child, mother, mother's sisters, mother's mother, and her mother who often constitute the family unit. Grandmother represents the stable figure, her daughters frequently having to work, sometimes at a distance, knowing that she can be depended upon to provide affection and good care of the children. Traditional women do not resent this role. Now that they are older, the younger women have assumed the more burdensome tasks of earning a livelihood, often the most difficult and tedious work, the only kind available. Older women now are able to turn their attentions to the young children. The great respect due these grandmothers is not likely to break down completely as this family form is replaced by the nuclear family.

Among the Navajo Indians of the Southwest, grandmother also represents a very highly respected figure. The Navajo reckon descent through the female line of the family, and it is the grandmother who generally maintains the shepherds' camp and the flocks, as well as assumes care of children for periods of time while the younger women and men engage in work, schooling, and travel. Modern Navajos frequently bring their children to grandmother's camp to learn the traditional culture and to learn to herd sheep.

And there are those women who, arriving as immigrants, still retain the traditions of their upbringing, and struggle to strike a happy balance between their desire to be included in the lives of their grandchildren and their realization that they must maintain a friendly distance or risk banishment by their own children. Off to visit grandmother's house, but only on Thanksgiving, may do in New England, but the infrequent visit can be a heartbreak to the woman of another tradition who expected to be a mother to the grandchild, as her grandmother was to her.

The greatest wrench of all occurs when grandparents are totally denied relationship to their grandchildren. And this can very well be the case in modern society as divorce rates go up and mothers, or fathers as the case may be, take the children, denying their in-laws rights. Usually in divorce cases, one or the other parent retains custody, with some visitation rights to the other. The rights of grandparents have not ordinarily been explicated, leaving the parties free to work things out informally. But these informal arrangements have sometimes been the cause of great anguish for grandparents who have been cut off from their children's children.

In 1976 one such situation came to the attention of the courts. The woman, a fifty-five-year-old grandmother, had not been permitted to see her only grandchild in more than three years. Her son had been divorced, and sometime later was killed in an automobile accident. At this point, the mother refused to allow his parents to see or communicate in any way with the child. The Appellate Division in Brooklyn, New York, ruled that ". . . visits with a grandparent are often a precious part of a child's experience." And in addition, the unanimous ruling stated: "Animosity between the mother of the children and their grandparents is not a proper basis for the denial of visitation privileges to the grandparents; nor is it a proper yardstick by which to measure the best interests of the children."

The court also cited a New Jersey court decision which held: "There are benefits which develop upon the grandchild from the relationship with his grandparents which he cannot derive from any other relationship. Neither the Legislature nor this court is blind to human truths which grandparents and grandchildren have always known."[15]

Experience around the grandparent role can be so varied. There are those women who, looking and feeling marvelous in their middle age, are proud to exclaim, "That's my grandchild!" Hardly the image of the gray-haired lady in apron and shawl, they revel in their attractiveness and accomplishment at now being, in addition to everything else they may be, grandmothers. Yet there are those who see in becoming grandmothers a mark of age, changed position, and resent the evidence that the years have passed. I recall one young woman, the mother of two handsome sons, who brought them with her to the department store where her mother worked. The grandmother, for no reason other than vanity, recoiled from the encounter. "Take them away," she said, "I don't want anyone to know I'm a grandmother." Needless to say this exaggerated reaction to the evidence of her age and changed generational status shocked her daughter.

In much of the world, *not* to have grandchildren is the tragedy: Not to have one's own descendants to love and care for, not to have one's own descendants to care for one as age progresses represents the worst eventuality.

And in some places this is institutionalized still further, for one's own descendants insure that the afterlife as well will be insured. Descendants were necessary to the traditional Buddhist Chinese to insure well-being in the afterlife—they were needed to perform the necessary rituals.

One of the eventualities for some modern American women is that they are likely never to become grandmothers. As mothering is devalued, and young people postpone marriage and even decide to do without children, life without grandchildren becomes a very real possibility. The courts have recognized that there are benefits to the grandchild which are derived from relationship with the grandparents. It could also be argued that there are benefits to the grandparents, Buddhists or not, that derive from relationships with grandchildren. An essential quality of life—the continuation of the species—a glimpse into the future, and the perpetuation of our wisdom comes with contact with our progeny. To lose that contact is to break the chain of survival.

## Daughter Role

Just as a woman, so long as she has children, never seems to give up mothering, so a woman, as long as her own mother or father live, never gives up being herself a daughter.

Ties to husband, children, career, or self-interest often take a woman long distances both in space and emotional ties from parents. But there is strong evidence that middle-aged women, particularly, take their daughter role seriously. They do feel responsibility for aging parents. They do provide financial assistance. Often, however, they are unable to provide all the emotional and physical nurture and attention that the older parent either requires or demands— separated by distance, education, beliefs, and other responsibilities as a wife and mother, and often worker, herself. Even where money might seem to ease matters, these responsibilities felt toward older parents are not necessarily eased, for the emotional needs of the aged are often greater than a woman can provide without affecting seriously other areas of her life. Total devotion is a full-time occupation. Providing nursing care when needed, overseeing medical attention, providing activities to ease loneliness are burdens that middle-aged daughters feel deeply toward parents.

While families were large and some members always about, the aged were not alone. Resolving her many responsibilities toward the generations above and below her, to herself, and her husband remains a major dilemma for the modern woman, for now the elderly are increasingly isolated, while remaining dependent. Individual women handle these situations differently and some feel greater responsibility—sometimes guilt—than others. But the problem of the aged is one that requires major attention by the whole society. The issues involved are greater than particular persons' interaction with each other, reflecting major social trends and problems.

## Wife Role

A wife is above all else a sex partner. Everywhere in the world where people marry, a husband expects to have sexual relations with his wife. Except for those places where it no longer matters or where particular men don't care, a wife is also expected to become a mother —to bear children. Barrenness has been a major cause of divorce in many places of the world and within many religious systems. And where there is no sexual consummation, marriage cannot be said to exist.

But a wife is many other things as well—throughout history and throughout the world she has also been an economic partner, tending the fields, managing the accounts, trading at the marketplace or, as in the present, working at the office or factory or school to augment or make her required—sometimes willing, other times reluctant —contribution to the needs of daily living.

But never before in the history of the world, as in our times, has a wife been required to be so many things to her husband. In other times and places, marriage partners tended to their tasks but sought their emotional ties and friendships, their amusements and comforts, from others. The modern wife plays all the roles shared by family and friends at other times. She must be friend, companion, lover, mistress, housekeeper, mother of children, accountant, nurse, worker, counselor, decorator, hostess, etc., etc., etc., all rolled into one. And, in addition, given the closeness with which a man and woman are thrust together in our monogamous marriages and small nuclear families, if any of these tasks prove incompatible with each other—scrubbing the kitchen floor may look glamorous when done on television, but hardly so in one's own kitchen and scarcely the picture of the lover-mistress; or mediating between their sometimes troublesome pre-adult children and their often irritable father; or if one job is done poorly or incompetently—the whole house of roles comes tumbling down. And as for the woman herself, some of these roles can cause enough friction for her to want out from the whole scene.

The pulls and tugs of a world that presents numerous images and choices of desirable women to men cannot help but create some questions, disappointments, problems, and threats to the monogamous marriage. There is one movement, appealing to those women who wish to maintain a traditional subordinate role in their marriage relationships with their husbands, that uses dress and grooming, role playing, and costume change to help accomplish this goal.

Over half a million American women have bought and may be responding to the message of the *Total Woman*, described by Marabel Morgan in her immensely successful book published in the early 1970s.[16] Followers of this movement are urged to surprise and titillate their husbands, keeping them happy and content and satisfied sexually by a variety of assignments and suggestions. "Eat by candlelight; you'll light his candle." Call him on the phone and tell him you crave his body. Dress in frilly and fancy nightgowns, stay far away from flannel. And to play the roles of all the potential romances and fantasies of his life—to keep him at home and interested in you—dress up in costumes to greet him when he returns from work, says Mrs. Morgan. "Your husband needs you to fulfill his daydreams. You can be lots of different women to him. Costumes provide variety without him ever leaving home."

In many ways, this advice appeals to those women who wish to continue their traditional roles while themselves playing at all the other people they might be, bringing the glamour and romance of the world portrayed in the mass media into their own living rooms.

Feminists would argue that this movement is a sham, deluding women into manipulative behavior to keep their husbands interested in them, while giving up much of themselves. But Total Woman advocates argue, "It is only when a woman surrenders her life to her husband, reveres and worships him, that she becomes truly beautiful to him." Mrs. Morgan also instructs that then ". . . she becomes a priceless jewel, the glory of femininity, his queen! . . . What if the king makes the wrong decision? . . . the queen is still to follow him." Appealing to religious belief she says, "You wives must submit to your husbands' leadership in the same way you submit to the Lord."

Now, the Total Woman movement may very well improve the spirit and tone of some listless marriages and give many women a new interest in their looks, households, husbands, and sex lives. But it could be argued that this total dedication to a narrowly defined feminine role, totally subordinate to a man and household, encourages a very limited set of interests and options for women as wives. And what is to happen to such women when they can no longer fulfill the roles of sex kitten and glamour girl as they grow older? Can playing at roles really replace more active participation in the world as children grow and leave home?

A similar view of wifely roles goes back to the pre-Civil War United States. A description of a wife in the ante bellum South, written in 1854, says:

> So long as she is nervous, fickle, capricious, delicate, diffident and dependent, man will worship and adore her. Her weakness is her strength, and her true art is to cultivate and improve that weakness. Woman naturally shrinks from public gaze and from the struggle and competition of life. . . . in truth, woman, like children, has but one right and that is the right to protection. The right to protection involves the obligation to obey. A husband, a lord and master, whom she should love, honor, and obey, nature designed for every woman. . . . If she be obedient she stands little danger of maltreatment.[17]

At the same time, these aristocratic Southern women were expected to be competent women, acting as hostesses, maintaining open houses, shining tables, and well-stocked wine cellars. They cared for their homes and children, took morning rides and were expected to "care for the souls and bodies of black people." And, in effect, the legislative and executive powers of the house—for these people a considerable enterprise—were in the hands of the women.

Still, women were expected to play the role of subservient wives. In good measure, the image of the submissive woman was reinforced by evangelical religious theory. It was based on the teachings of St. Paul who stressed that men found intelligence in women a quality that in general distressed rather than pleased.

It is the same view of the inherent inferiority of the wife, subservient to her husband, which, in fact, is subverted by women into pretense and manipulation—acting the part but in effect controlling the relationship. This point of view is basic to the very popular Total Woman movement in the United States. Many of the women who adhere to the ideology of the Total Woman are actually working wives, important in economic life and highly intelligent. Still they virtually reinforce the notion that marks them as inferior to their husbands.

## Housewife Role

In an extraordinary study based on interviews with London women, sociologist Ann Oakley turned her attention to an examination of the role of housewife.[18] It really is interesting to note that this role, played by so many women and valued or devalued as the case may be by society, has, until recently, received such minimal attention by social scientists. Dr. Oakley's study fills a gap in our knowledge and understanding.

The women of London reacted differently to different aspects of the role of housewife. The most valued quality of being a housewife was the autonomy of the role—the right to do your own thing pretty much as and when you wished. Housewives work on their own time, they punch no clock, they are their own boss. They enjoy getting out of the house and meeting people, shopping, etc. The role of consumer is valued. The thing they enjoy least is the housework they must do. They perceive cleaning the house especially as having low status. It is monotonous and lonely. On the other hand, cooking, shopping, and washing are not disliked so much. Women, however, tend to set their own routines at home, maintain their own standards, and derive satisfaction from a job well done, a well-kept house. They dislike the cleaning but enjoy the results. However, the trouble with housecleaning is that the house is bound to get dirty or unkempt again, and the whole process has to be repeated—housework is a job never done! These London housewives worked an average of seventy-seven hours a week—some worked as much as one hundred five.

Although outside employment could offer company, social recognition, and financial reward, many women preferred the autonomy of being housewives. Especially among the working-class women, there is a strong motivation to declare a personal identification with domesticity, and this, in turn, leads to a search for satisfaction in housework.

It's hardly necessary to go to London to recognize that many women at home would not trade their roles for the time clock of factory or office. For the woman in higher status jobs, the switch may be desirable. The fact is, most women who work outside the home do so because they have to. For many of these women the loss of autonomy associated with working in a factory or office, subject to imposed routines, beholden to employer and superiors, represents a poor substitute for the autonomous life led by most women in the housewife role.

But there is still another reason many women prefer to be housewives. And that is that to be a housewife for many, especially the kinds of women studied by Dr. Oakley, including the working-class women of modern London, is so consonant with what they regard as being appropriately feminine.

There is a combination of factors that makes for including "housewife" within the world of traditional femininity. Marriage, motherhood, and housewife often go together. And girls are easily socialized for domesticity and the adult performance of the housewife role and those other social arrangements with which housewives are associated. Women learn to think of the housewife role as "natural" and, while not pleased with all aspects of it, make efforts to derive satisfaction from the role. Whether they like it or not, they believe they should enjoy being housewives.

And the competent housewife, fulfilling her role with skill and satisfaction, is valued in many cultures about the world as the ideal of femininity, the fulfillment of the role of woman. The Yiddish language has a word for such a woman, she is a *balabusta*. And wherever women are permitted to choose brides for their sons, whatever other abilities the girl may need, skill and industry in housekeeping are ordinarily among them.

A cultural system, however, that completely encapsulates women within the world of marriage, motherhood, and domesticity, with little opportunity to perform other roles, makes any dissatisfaction with it appear to be abnormal to some extent. Often women are not permitted to state their discontent openly, and when they do they are vilified in some way. The "nagging" wife, the "irritable mother," yes, even the "ball breaker." Sometimes a woman conceals dissatisfaction even from herself, having been raised to believe it normal to be happy and content in the housewife role, especially if it is defined as the only appropriate feminine role. Psychosomatic illness, fatigue, and depression, even the image of the hysterical woman, are frequently the expression of discontent with the imposed and internalized acceptance of the role of housewife.

Dr. Oakley points out, with great insight, that the conventional psychoanalytic explanation of the troubled housewife is a little more profound, but hence a little more dangerous. The unsatisfied housewife now becomes the unsatisfied wife and/or the maladjusted mother, and what becomes necessary for a cure is adaptation and adjustment to the resented role.

"Housewives' disease" is a recognized medical syndrome, associated with depression. Unfortunately, the sociocultural reason for the depression—the insistence of the culture upon defining femininity in terms of the limited range of housewife, mother, and wife—is thus neglected in favor of medical solutions, tranquilizers, estrogen, or psychoanalysis.

Not all women in modern society feel that marriage, motherhood, and domesticity represent their only possible roles in the society. They do not accept the common cultural attitudes that attempt to impose guilt, suspicion, and resentment toward women who have insisted, whether by necessity or choice, that they be involved in the larger society outside their homes without losing their femininity as a result. But they are up against constant reminders. Is she working because she can't get a man to marry her? Is she unmarried or turned on to "Women's Lib" because she's a Lesbian? Doesn't her husband satisfy her—is that why she looks for satisfaction outside the home? What's the matter with her husband? Can't he support her?

When a man tries to get ahead he's labeled ambitious; a woman doing the same is labeled aggressive. When a man makes more money than his wife he's admired and considered responsible; when a wife makes more money than her husband and is responsible, she's out to wear the pants. When a man is viewed as ambitious, successful, and of high status, he is honored, valued, and respected. His wife is considered fortunate. When a woman is ambitious and successful, she is considered dissatisfied, unhappy, neurotic, and her husband often belittled rather than admired.

Fortunately, in our heterogeneous culture, more than one set of values and attitudes pervades. Accomplished women are admired, our laws expound equality, and neither all women nor all men are now limited by a completely restricted view of what it is to be a woman and a wife.

Fifty-three per cent of American women do work outside the home and are familiar with roles outside the home. It is, of course, difficult to tell how many of them are conflicted by so doing. The reality is that there is often conflict, especially given the nuclear family, the high rate of divorce, and the frequent absence of any kinsmen to look after children. The conflict extends to the working woman whose husband retains another value system, not helping with the housekeeping. Often the woman who is encouraged to seek employment outside the home to "calm her nerves," "take her mind off herself and her troubles," as if work were the therapy for the illness of the depressed or discontented housewife, finds she has traded one set of chores for a situation in which she now has her housekeeping plus another job as well.

Somebody has to do the housekeeping, unless we all join the Mad Hatter's tea party and simply move on to another place as soon as our own becomes untidy. With non-biodegradable plastic bags and aluminum cans, we can't even do that for long before the whole world becomes one big garbage heap. There can be little quarrel with the need to keep house, nor with those women who choose to make it their life's work. It must be recognized, however, that, by the same token, for some women to derive their identity from only the roles associated with domesticity, thereby denying them the open expression of the discontent that may inevitably arise for many, trouble is bound to arise.

Women are valued for many other roles in many places in the world. Housecleaning and other household chores are sometimes the tasks of the young children or the very old women, and sometimes, as is increasingly the case among ourselves, they involve the men. There is no one solution to the problem of who is to take out the garbage. However, whoever it is, hopefully, does not derive his or her sense of masculinity or femininity from the task.

Some women find that the nicest aspects of their roles as house-keepers get lost to them around middle age. With their children grown and off, they may feel more autonomous than ever—no more dirty socks to pick up from the floor, less laundry, fewer chops to broil for dinner, and fewer idiosyncratic appetites to satisfy. But then comes husband's retirement.

Some women then find that their household responsibilities in-crease timewise and their autonomy decreases. With husband in the house, it is neither romantic nor appropriate to be on the telephone with girl friends all morning, with time later to do the beds and the dishes. Hair up in curlers, cream on the face, nightrobe still on were O.K. while he was at work—plenty of time to get dressed later at your leisure; now he's there to see you at all hours. And then there is lunch. If you don't have it with him, who will?

Many retired men who previously had little to do with the house-keeping do try to help. Studies have indicated that when they do they often take over the very task that the housewife had found a most desirable part of *her* responsibility—shopping. Shopping had meant contact with the outside world, opportunity to meet people, to engage in conversation, to dress for the public appearance. These are precisely the areas most comfortable for retired men whose wives had been fully responsible for housekeeping earlier.

Retirement of a husband presents special conditions for many a middle-aged wife who, until that point in her husband's career, was accustomed to routines that included the husband being away from the house much of the time, as well as his being occupied with activities and friends that affected the social and financial life of the couple. In modern society, where so much of a man's status, posi-tion, and prestige are dependent upon the job he holds within the economic order, to be cut off from that is bound to create shifts in life style and relationships within the family as well.

There is no one way that men respond to retirement, unless it could be said that all experience a change in status and a readjust-ment of activity. They are not all about to have heart attacks and die either. The occasional story of people dying soon after retirement neglects to mention that frequently people do not retire until they are too ill to work. Retirement generally comes at later ages as well. American men, for example, although retirement ages are dropping, tend to relate retirement to the age of sixty-two to sixty-five because of the Social Security System. For many, this is the dangerous decade in terms of life expectancy, so the association between retirement and death seems to hold, whereas it is really the association between age and life expectancy.

The adjustment made by retired couples seems to be closely related to whether the couple is free to enjoy life together with minimal responsibility for others, as well as their financial ability to deal with retirement—after all, retirement means the ending of the usual income for most people. Sociologist Alan C. Kerkoff did an analysis of 135 white retired couples in the North Carolina-Virginia area.[19] He found what might be expected, that those couples who enjoyed their retirement most were, in general, relatively nucleated; that is, they were independent units with minimal dependence on their children as well as with independence from and minimal responsibility for their own parents. They were couples who maintained a functioning, home-based pattern of life.

One of the factors that was found to be related to the level of morale of the couple had to do with participation in household tasks. Morale was higher when the man participated! Having a man around all the time without his helping is no bargain for some women. Perhaps the complaint "I married him for better or worse but not for lunch" is best answered by husband's helping with the dishes.

Mutual support activities with children also made for higher morale—but demands and dependence on children did not. It's nice to learn you can depend on your grown children—but better not to need them.

Retirement does not mean the same thing for all social classes. As the experience of London housewives indicates, and the Kerkoff study also showed, women in the working-class groups are used to doing the housework, their husbands resenting that role. Men at retirement begin to take on some of the tasks, such as shopping, even looking forward to them, but sense the conflict between their actual behavior and what they believe proper for a man. Couples have to work out these tensions. For many, the first five years of retirement provide the greatest satisfaction. After five years, many retirees become restive and wish to return to activity in the world outside the home.

Social class, both because of possible differences in values and preparation for other activities, and because of the money to enjoy retirement, affected the kinds of responses found in the Kerkoff study. Upper-level persons of the professional and managerial class did not particularly welcome retirement. This is understandable—if one's position in society has a high value placed upon it, and therefore upon you, to give it up is to possibly lose a great deal. Also, many such people enjoy their careers. Yet it is precisely the people of this class who have the best experience with retirement. Perhaps they have the best pensions and probably the most money saved. They usually have more education and resources to enjoy other aspects of life besides work, for example, study, travel, etc. Middle-level persons, white collar workers, and skilled workers welcomed retirement but had less favorable reactions to it. Lower-level groups were more passive about retirement, but responded more negatively to it. Many of these families are less nucleated than those of the upper classes, with more interdependence among relatives. There are often children and grandchildren dependent, competing for the affections and attention of the spouse, creating tensions for a man around the house.

## Magic and Religious Roles

In many societies, magic and religious roles, such as those of diviner, priest, religious teacher, etc., are not open to women except after they have reached menopause. In part, this opening up of the more prestigious powerful roles associated with magic and religion is due to the ending of menstruation. In almost all societies, the blood associated with menstruation inspires some fear—menstruating women are considered "impure," and contact with such women considered a defilement. In many societies menstruating women are secluded from the males, and frequently sexual intercourse forbidden with them, their presence considered a defilement. The traditional Hebrew custom of the ritual bath, or Mikvah, required for women twelve days after the beginning of their menstruation, illustrates a ceremonial purification enabling the woman to resume marital relations without danger of contaminating her husband. This is not always the case, however. Indeed, among the glamour- and youth-oriented natives of the Marquesas in the South Pacific, a cure for prolonged menstrual bleeding was intercourse with the household head!

In those societies with strict menstrual taboos, with the menopause women are freed from the defiling presence of menstruation. They are now considered safe for ceremonial purposes. In many places, it is only after menopause, for example, that women are free to conduct the ceremonials around childbirth, marriage, and puberty. It is now that they can be midwives and can participate in the religious rituals of the group.

## Women in Government

Women have not ordinarily played very important roles within modern governments. This largely reflects the lower status women have in male-dominated societies. But this hardly means that women cannot or do not fulfill the duties and responsibilities of political leadership in the modern world, or in the traditional world of other societies.

There is the stereotype prejudice against women in government—they are thought to be emotional, undependable, their menstrual cycles lead to rule by hormones rather than the rational mind. The condition, it is believed, is not improved by menopause, when again the notion of rule by the endocrine glands is believed to induce women into irrational and dangerous behavior.

What utter nonsense! Women's lack of participation as political leaders is a function of history and social structure. In the United States today, the evidence of the way in which there exists both subtle and obvious methods for keeping women out of important roles in government is being increasingly exposed. The Civil Rights Legislation of the past decade has prompted legal action in this direction. For example, in 1976 a suit filed in the U. S. District Court of Washington, D.C., claimed discrimination in "all aspects of the personnel system" of the U. S. State Department's diplomatic corps, in regard to hiring, promotion, and assignments. As a result of the suit, the Department issued data concerning the employment of women. They said that 312 women make up 9 per cent of the Foreign Service Officer Corps numbering 3,461 individuals. Clearly, women are not in important positions in significant numbers in these more influential roles. Still, the figures represent an increase of 3 per cent within the decade 1966–76.[20]

During the past forty years, there have been seven women career diplomats who have served as United States ambassadors. This number is likely to increase in the future as more women are nominated for these prestigious posts.

Senior positions in government around the world usually go to older men and women. It takes years to develop the experience, establish the relationships, and the evidence of ability that the senior positions usually require. Of course, there are positions that in some societies are inherited, and age is incidental. But in societies where one's abilities to rule, or one's access to a high position, is either bought or earned by performance or the wisdom and knowledge that come with experience, it is likely to take living into middle age before reaching the top.

Those societies that value the role of middle-aged women as participators in government and give women the opportunity to actively participate in government are those in which the status of these women does not decline as a result of growing older. Indira Gandhi and Golda Meir, who have played significant roles in the important affairs of their countries and the world, symbolize the relatively high position of women at mid-life in the contemporary Hindu society of India and the modern State of Israel. The particular political philosophies and actions of these two leaders might be criticized by contenders, but their rule and judgments are not attributed to glands and gender.

And among the traditional societies, there are also many in which women take on the important role of governors at menopause. Among the Lovedu of Africa, for example, in addition to being the romantic consorts of younger men, older women have important political power. They are ruled by a queen, as well, whose function it is to make the rain—the necessary condition for well-being. It would be the height of incomprehensibility to argue among such peoples that women are not competent to rule simply by virtue of being women.[21]

In West Africa, the biological capabilities for childbearing mark women as especially strong and active agents in society, capable of holding high political office. Among the Mende of Sierra Leone, for example, women have enjoyed high offices as lineage heads, heads of secret societies, and as chiefs for centuries. In their maturity they continue to enjoy the respect and following of the younger people.[22]

Women as leaders in government are likely to, indeed are entitled to, make the same human errors as men. There is really little reason to assume that there is something magical or mystical about women solving the problems of the world. As human beings, products of their society, they generally share with the men common attitudes and values. Once the same education, opportunity to be involved in social interaction, and experience are available to them, their actions are likely to be similar. The world did not change when women got the vote! The fact is, however, that exclusion affects the choices, opportunities, and the prestige of women.

Having arrived at menopause, the removal of women from the overt sexuality of menstruation and childbearing enables women of many societies to appear like the men, removed from many of the taboos and restrictions of their childbearing years. This does not mean removal from sexual liaisons with men—the Lovedu are a case in point—but it does mean that the woman at menopause is free to participate where she had previously been excluded. The Civil Rights Legislation in the United States seems to be performing the same function for all women, at all ages.

# Menopause—When

On Melville Island, Northern Australia, there live a group of people called the Tiwi. Among Tiwi women, it is believed that the gradual stopping or complete cessation of sexual intercourse is the cause of menopause.[1]

If the Tiwi women were correct, sex and more sex would be the prescription of choice to keep women menstruating forever. But life is not so simple, and the fact is that with or without sex, menopause is a universal fact of life for all women who survive through their fifties, with only the rarest of women continuing to menstruate beyond that time.

## When Does Menopause Occur?

Menopause, the end of the monthly periods, can occur at any age after the onset of menstruation due to natural developmental changes in women. However, early cessation of the menses is not common although it does occur normally. The vast majority of women cease menstruation during the decade of forty-five to fifty-five years of age, with most around the age of fifty to fifty-two. In occasional women, normal menstruation continues until much later and rare pregnancies are known to have occurred past the middle fifties.

It really is not possible, at present, for a woman to know exactly when she personally will stop menstruating, although, since genetic inheritance seems to play a role in determining her age of menopause, her family history might give her some general clues, especially if there is a history of particularly early or late menopause. Knowing that history, however, is no guarantee to her of the number of years in which childbearing is possible, a factor that might influence a woman's decision concerning the postponement of motherhood.

To the medical community, the normal age of menopause has always been of keen interest, but for reasons far more concerned with the physical health of women. Ordinarily there are two normal reasons for menstruation to cease. One obviously is pregnancy—bleeding during pregnancy is not a healthy condition, and by definition the loss of the uterine lining which occurs with menstruation effectively aborts the usual pregnancy. The second normal reason for cessation of menses is the menopause itself, which marks the end of the cyclical preparation of the uterus for the reception of a fertilized ovum.

Until modern, sophisticated techniques such as hormone assays, X rays, and biopsies to study tissues, etc., were developed, it was a problem for physicians to make a determination of whether or not the ending of the menses was due to the natural course of a woman's development, or whether it was due to some pathological condition, such as a tumor, for example. For this reason, as well as because of their great curiosity concerning the nature of mankind, physicians throughout history have paid some attention to the matter of determining the normal age of menopause for women.

The great philosophers and physicians of classical Greece and Rome, including Aristotle, Diocles, physicians of the Hippocratic school, Pliny, Soranus, Oribasius, Aetilus, and Paulua Aegineta, wrote on the age of menopause. Their works extended from the fourth century B.C. to the sixth century A.D. Aristotle wrote: "Generally speaking, for the most part . . . fifty marks the limit to the capacity of reproduction in women." Pliny, the Elder (first century A.D.) wrote in his *Historia Naturalis*: "A woman does not bear children after the age of fifty, and with the majority menstruation ends at forty."[2]

The writers of classical Greece and Rome were interested in questions that are still of interest today, such as, whether or not there is any relation between the age at which menstruation begins and the age at which it ends, or whether there is any connection between a woman's body build and the age of menopause. On the whole, these classical writers generally state an age range of forty to fifty for menopause with an upward limit of sixty often cited, little different from the current picture.

Physicians in medieval Europe continued this interest in the normal age of menopause, and again the most commonly mentioned age of menopause cited during this period was fifty. One remarkable woman of the twelfth century, Hildegard of Bingen, who founded a convent and wrote extensively on medical matters, wrote: ". . . the menses cease in women from the fiftieth year and sometimes in certain ones from the sixtieth. . . . Sometimes it rarely happens that the occasional woman from any super fluidity whatsoever with difficulty conceives a single time even up to the eightieth year."[3]

It is interesting that on the whole these early observers of the course of female development appear to agree with contemporary studies, which place menopause, on the average in Europe, as a little over fifty years. In the Netherlands one study reports an average age of 51.4, for example. In England another study reports an average age of 50.8. South African data is similar.[4]

Has menopause been occurring later in the lives of women?

The evidence from the classical writers is not enough, by itself, to answer the question of whether or not the age of menopause has been pushed upward in recent times due perhaps to better health and care, or whether it has remained the same throughout history. There is not enough data on samples or method of study from the ancient sources, although they clearly point to a similar age. The question itself is an important as well as interesting one, for if the age of menopause is growing later and later, that could have important effects on our lives. It would mean a prolongation of the child-bearing potential of women. It might even imply that the aging process is not inevitable, but due to conditions in the environment which provoke early decline.

The question is difficult to answer with assurance for a number of reasons. One, the determination of actual menopause is not a simple matter, and, second, it is difficult to compare results of research studies one with the other. For example, some studies simply accept the report of women that they have stopped menstruating. But others take into account the fact that at least twelve calendar months should go by without a period for menopause actually to have occurred. Since some women skip a period or two and then resume menstruation, for them to report they have stopped before they begin again clearly influences the age results. Many studies are based on women's memories, and since menopause is hardly the startling event that a first menstruation is, again estimates may affect results, especially among women who are unaccustomed to paying close attention to calendars but measure time instead by events or seasons, as do many in the world. Also, some studies suffer from the fact that they include results from women who have stopped menstruating but do not include those women who continue to menstruate and would therefore be reporting a later age.

The current knowledge concerning the question of whether or not menopause is occurring at later ages indicates that the conditions of modern life are *not* making any significant changes in the age of menopause. The question remains an open one, however, for we cannot know the answer with certainty until there is far more research that would have to first of all define menopause age clearly—for example, one year past last menstrual period; and follow groups of women longitudinally, i.e., throughout the whole period of their reproductive lives or even longer, in order to get data on actual menstrual and menopause symptomology. These studies would have to take into account many variables including the socioeconomic status of the women studied, their general health, occupation, where they live, their marital status, number of children, ethnic and racial background, etc.

For the time being, the evidence is overwhelmingly in favor of the understanding that the age of menopause seems to have been fairly constant throughout recorded history. The implications of this are far reaching. This implies that menopause occurs in the natural development of woman from birth through death, and that it follows the inexorable dictates of some internal time clock which comes to us in the genes of the human species.

Menopause seems to be somewhat different from menarche, or the onset of menstruation, which has changed insofar as age of occurrence is concerned. Careful studies by Tanner and others have indicated that the age of onset of menstruation has been moving steadily downward in Europe and America among Caucasians during the last one hundred years.[5] The decline was three to four months every decade between 1845 and 1960, to what is currently an average of thirteen years. Of course, this is only an average, and individual girls are known to begin menstruation normally anywhere within the range of ten to eighteen—even a generation ago, in the United States, the manufacturers of sanitary napkins promoted the sale of the pamphlet *Marjorie's 12th Birthday*. The European and American age of menstruation is in contrast to one of the slowest developmental rates ever reported among some natives of New Guinea, where the average age of onset of menstruation is eighteen.[6] Earlier or later menstruation within the accepted range of ten to eighteen among Western girls can be perfectly normal and need not necessarily provoke anxiety about precocious or delayed development.

But while many were cheering what seemed to be the accelerated rate of development of girls in the advanced industrial countries, with most of the credit given to better food, improved sanitation and health conditions, it was also fairly obvious that the age of onset of menstruation could not keep going down and down and down. The notion of the baby girl capable of reproduction is a contradiction to the characteristics of mankind which require a capable mother caring for an infant through a prolonged childhood. The very nature of the species includes a period of development into maturity after birth. None of us springs full-blown from our mother's womb like so many Athenas from the head of Zeus. And, as if to emphasize this point, recent studies in the United States indicate that the average age of first menstruation has stopped going down.

Even should we find that improved health and living conditions lead to an increase in the fertility span for women from ages thirteen to fifty-three to twelve to fifty-five, we might ask, so what? Just as fertility in the infant is not necessarily desirable, so most women past fifty are not particularly eager to experience childbearing and child raising. Besides, it is horrifying to think of the disastrous consequences to mankind if each of 2,000,000,000 females exercised even her current biological potential of permitting each of some 30,000 to 400,000 ovarian follicles from developing into a human being. Our current world population would escalate at a dizzying pace from its current 4,000,000,000 to 60,000,000,000,000 up to 800,000,000,000,-000. It is fortunate that our very genes prevent such a catastrophe.

As it is, a reproductive span averaging around thirty-five years does not usually produce vast numbers of offspring anyway. One of the most fertile women in history was Maria Christian, who was the daughter of Fletcher Christian, of the ship *Bounty,* and his Polynesian wife. Maria was the mother of twenty-five children. Few women on earth have had as many. The explanation for her fertility does not lie in any prolongation of the childbearing years—just that she regularly became pregnant while she could.

## Relationship between Age of First Menstruation and Menopause

Many women have wondered whether or not there is any relationship between the age at which they began to menstruate and the age at which they would experience menopause. There seems to be a logic that argues that if menstruation begins relatively early, and that since this represents what appears to be a pattern of rapid development, this pattern would then bring on an early menopause. There is another logic that would argue that early menstruation represents better health and vitality, and continuing health and vitality would therefore bring on a late menopause. Does a later first menstruation mean a later menopause, or does it mean an earlier one? Does an early first menstruation mean an early menopause or a later one?

All of the above positions seem to have *no* relationship to reality. Women whose menopause comes at fifty, for example, include those who began menstruating at various ages. In order to conclusively prove this point, it is necessary to study the histories of women, not only from their memories, but over the course of their lives. One such study was made. In the 1920s Dr. Alan E. Treloar enrolled a group of University of Minnesota freshman co-eds, whose first menstruations were documented (they were young enough and calendar-conscious enough to give their first menstruation dates accurately), and these women were followed up over forty years through the present. Using great caution, Dr. Treloar considered that menopause had occurred only after *two* calendar years had passed since the last menstruation. On the basis of the evidence of these women's menstrual histories, he concluded that there was no correlation between the age at which menstruation started and the age at which it came to an end.[7]

This study also showed that the length of a woman's menstrual life ranged from twenty-two to forty-five years, an average of 35.9 years; figures far more variable than the range of years during which women reach menopause.

## Geography and Menopause

Another question that has been of interest to women and those who study them has been whether or not the place where one lives has any effect on menopause. Of particular interest has been the question of altitude. Altitude is known to have some significant effects on the human physiology, so it seemed likely that altitude would also affect menopause. Several researchers have attempted to answer this question. While their results are interesting, it must be kept in mind that many of these studies were made among women where record keeping is poor; the definitions of menopause varied; and, these were not studies that followed the same groups of women over a period of years. These factors force us to exercise caution concerning their conclusions, but nonetheless, the results are highly suggestive and certainly warrant further investigation of the question. What has been found? It appears that altitude does have an influence on the age of menopause.

In one study, 483 women of the Rajput caste in India were examined to determine the effect of altitude. Two hundred forty-three of the women lived at low altitude (984 feet or 300 meters above sea level). The remaining 240 lived at middle altitude (6,562–8,202 feet or 2,000–2,500 meters above sea level). Perhaps most significantly, the researcher reports that few women had any difficulty with menopause at either altitude. As far as age at menopause was concerned, the women at middle altitude were about a year lower than the age of women at low altitude.[8]

The results of this study support one made in the Andes mountains in South America, where it was found that women who lived at high altitudes, above 10,000 feet, experienced menopause one and one-half years earlier than women at low altitude.[9]

The explanation for these results is still only suggestive. It is hypothesized that hypoxia, or oxygen deprivation at the higher altitudes, creates stresses on the body that reduce the steroid hormone levels at an earlier age, thereby shortening the reproductive cycle. But the question has not been studied adequately for a definitive answer.

The implications of these studies concerning the effect of altitude on menopause are significant, but they need not cause the woman in Denver, Colorado, to assume that her menopause will come earlier than that of her friend living on the New Jersey shore. There is data that for every one hundred feet above sea level, age at menstruation is postponed three months, but the evidence for menopause is far from clear, and other factors, such as family history, affect the specific course of the individual woman's reproductive life.

It is known that airline stewardesses, working at high altitudes in pressurized cabins, do experience some menstrual irregularity. Now that, in the United States at least, there are antidiscrimination laws against age bias in hiring, it would be interesting to follow the menstrual histories through menopause of those women who remain flying until later ages. Investigation on the effect of air travel on this aspect of a woman's physiology should be of interest to all women who fly frequently.

Aside from altitude, does where a woman lives make any difference in her age of menopause? A 1966 study of women in the United States seems to indicate that for this country the difference, if any, is very minimal, measured in months, and not even that if one takes into account the possibility of statistical error. Thus, in the Northeast the mean age of menopause is 50.09; in the South, 50.05; and in the West, 49.97.[10]

Location may not make a significant difference—what about climate? Does living in the tropics make for an earlier or later menopause than living in the temperate zone? There are a number of old studies claiming that tropical climates retard menopause. Yet there are others claiming that in hot countries women age earlier and get their menopause earlier. The question of the relationship between climate and age of menopause awaits far more sophisticated research than that which has as yet been done. For the time being the question remains unanswered satisfactorily.

## Other Factors

A woman's social and economic class seems to be related, at least statistically, to an increased age at menopause. Some investigators have maintained that working-class women had an earlier menopause than women of upper-income levels. One 1959 study argued that better economic conditions and a normal diet delayed the age of menopause.[11] In 1966 MacMahon and Worcester studied over 3,500 women in the United States. They found that the women of higher income had a later menopause, also that urban women had a later menopause compared to rural women.[12] There seems to be little argument with the notion that improved living conditions permit a woman to live out the potential of her reproductive life span, but it would not justify the expectation that the prolongation can continue indefinitely.

There are still other factors to be considered in relation to the age of menopause. Does the number of children a woman has borne, for example, affect the age? Does the spacing of the children, or whether or not she nurses them and for how long a period affect the age of menopause? Here, once again, we are faced with contradictory evidence claimed by various investigators to answer these questions.

One of the early gynecologists to write on the subject, Currier, in 1897, believed that a series of childbirths and lactation (breast feeding) were the forerunners of menopause.[13] Later, Kisch and Stopes, writing in 1928 and 1936 respectively, claimed the opposite. Kisch maintained that women who had had three or more children, the last between the ages of thirty-eight and forty, would have the latest menopause.[14] Stopes claimed that nursing postpones the menopause and that childbearing might postpone it.[15] Indeed, during the period their works received attention, there was a belief among women that childbearing around the age of forty would postpone menopause and perpetuate youthfulness and health. Whether the preponderance of this idea influenced these writers, or whether or not they influenced the women is hard to determine. At any rate, since we know that menopause occurs up through the fifties, it is difficult to give childbirth or nursing the credit for a later menopause among women who bore children later, precisely because they were capable of doing so. In other words, it is difficult to claim a cause-and-effect relationship since those with earlier menopause would not have been able to have later children anyway.

Another study of women in Australia claimed that the menses ended later among women who had had a large number of pregnancies. Sixty-four per cent of those women without children ceased menstruating before the age of fifty, while only 37 per cent of those with five or more children did the same. Here, too, unfortunately, there is no record of the women's gynecological history, and it is difficult to determine whether or not the sample of women without children included those with gynecological difficulties.[16]

These questions, too, still remain incompletely investigated. For the time being, the evidence does not justify a continuous cycle of pregnancy and nursing to replace the recently discredited estrogen as a technique for staving off the disappearance of menstruation.

## Sex Activity and the Age of Menopause

One of the more interesting questions remaining is whether or not there is any relationship between a woman's sex-life history and her age of menopause. Do the Tiwi know something we don't? Yet, surprisingly, although this one has received plenty of attention from the moralizers, it has received relatively little serious scientific attention.

Sex and age do receive attention in cultures, however, and several mythologies about sex do exist. There are some men, for example, who believe that they have a finite allotment of semen to expend in their lifetimes. In order to preserve their virility they dole out semen sparingly, fearing that too frequent intercourse will sap them of their strength and that their sex ability will end early as a result. Some Yogas of India even practice what they claim is the ability to ejaculate and then reabsorb their semen.

This misguided notion has its counterpart in some beliefs about women and their sexual activity. Fortunately, current fashion does not support the point of view taught in Victorian sex manuals, which attributed menopausal woes to the expression of feminine passion, and which encouraged women to restrain their desire for sexual activity except for the purpose of becoming pregnant.

To emphasize the myriad adjustments made by mankind to the problem of understanding his condition, the Tiwi women believe that it is the very absence of sexual intercourse that brings on menopause! While Kinsey and Masters and Johnson do not discuss the age of menopause, they do argue that continued and regular intercourse are related to continued elasticity and lubrication of the vagina.

One study of 646 gynecological cases in an Israeli hospital found that earlier menopause occurred among single women. But it is difficult to conclude from this study whether these women had an earlier menopause because of absence of or limited sexual activity, or whether it was related to absence of childbearing, or whether some other factors explained the difference.[17]

A woman's sexual history may of course have some effects on her gynecological history where she has been exposed to serious infection or injury. But in the case of normally healthy women, whose occasional infections have been cleared up with good medical care, there is no evidence that sexual intercourse per se has any cause-and-effect relationship with the age of menopause.

The belief of Tiwi women that the ending of sexual intercourse is the cause of menopause, however, is related to their actual experience. Tiwi girls are married to very much older husbands before they have their first menstrual period. Indeed, their marriage contracts are arranged at birth, but they are not given over to their husbands until they are almost pubescent. It is believed that the sexual activities of that husband cause the girl to "grow up" and to begin menstruating. Throughout her life, the Tiwi woman is likely to be married to a succession of younger men, sometimes two or more, as her elderly husbands die. In addition, she is likely to have a number of extramarital sexual relationships, for Tiwi men are not given their brides until late in life and therefore seek liaisons with married women for their sexual satisfaction.

By the time she reaches menopause, a Tiwi woman is usually married to a relatively young man. At the same time, since this is a society in which a man may have several wives, she may now also be the oldest wife, and less favored as a sexual partner by her husband. In addition, she is less likely to have extramarital lovers for her lovers are by now old enough to marry. It has been suggested that this combination of factors—relative age of the wife among co-wives, fewer extramarital affairs, plus the likelihood that the husband will now be a young man with greater interest in younger wives—may be the reason Tiwi women say that "stopping of sexual intercourse causes menopause."

In any event, the Tiwi do not seem to regard sexual behavior among the elderly as improper, and indeed, to remain a widow is to lose a certain amount of "face," since the Tiwi regard it as normal for a woman to be contracted in marriage from the time she is born until the time she dies. When a woman reaches menopause she is not considered to be at the end of her life, indeed, her power and prestige are likely to increase. The Tiwi do recognize that postmenopausal women have a special status, but this time of life is different from the one yet to come—old age.

It is possible, but nowhere demonstrated, that there is a psychosomatic component to the age of menopause, and given a particular attitude toward sex, continued intercourse or its absence might cause an earlier or later menopause. For the time being, it does not seem that the prescription of the Tiwi women for continued sexual intercourse to postpone menopause would work. Would that it did—it would be the most delightful medicine of all.

All the factors discussed above have some bearing on the average age of menopause. For the individual woman, however, the most significant factors concerning her age at menopause are her own particular hereditary pattern of growth and development, as well as her own gynecological history. There are so many factors that influence the course of an individual's life, that age prediction at the present state of knowledge isn't possible. The chances are pretty good, though, that, given the known distribution of ages at menopause, the vast majority of women can anticipate continuation of their menstrual cycles, and their ability to conceive and bear a child until the period of their lives between forty-five and the early fifties.

# VIII

# Menopause—A Biological "Change of Life"

## THE PHYSIOLOGICAL FACTS

The word menopause means, simply, the cessation of menses, the end of the monthly periods. But there are peculiar contradictions in discussions about menopause. On the one hand, it is frequently talked about and discussed as if it happens all at once, and that it is simply a sudden biological event. Yet, general folk wisdom speaks of going through a "change of life" or the "changes," implying both that it is a process that takes time and that more than just biology is involved. Significant transitions—"changes"—between one or another stage of life are implied. Thus, menopause is seen as hardly a simple occurrence, but rather a process, both biological and social in nature.

As a biological event, menopause is a process, over time, of changing ovarian function and endocrine hormonal balance, eventually expressing itself as complete ending of menstruation and ability to conceive, facts that cannot be taken for granted until at least one calendar year has passed since the last menstruation.[1] Unfortunately, however, there is much confusion in both the popular and even medical literature dealing with the biological menopause. Women of forty and women up to age sixty-five are frequently lumped together as being menopausal. Yet the physical changes occurring in women ten or more years after they have arrived at menopause are scarcely the same as those physical changes seen in women within the decade preceding their final menstruation.

The body does not seem to change abruptly. Menopause does not mean that young women become old overnight. Women differ widely in their condition of health and vigor throughout life. There is, however, a universal biological experience shared by all women who live long enough, and that is the end of menstruation, menopause. And for some women there is also the experience of the "hot flush" or "sweats" which occasionally follow the close of the child-bearing period. What are these signs of menopause, and what do they mean?

## Symptoms of the Menopause

Classic signs that menopause is nearing or has arrived are irregularities or cessation of the menstrual periods. For some women, regular menstruation continues to take place during the years of their reproductive cycle until it suddenly stops, not to appear again. For other women, however, the pattern can be quite different. For several years before the actual end of menstruation, there can be a wide variety of menstrual patterns.

The changed patterns can include the absence of periods (amenorrhea); reduced frequency of menstruation, with cycles of longer than thirty-eight days (oligomenorrhea); lessened flow or shortening of the duration of the period (hypomenorrhea); or irregular or excessive bleeding during periods (menometrorrhagia).

If women become anxious, nervous, worried by these symptoms, these are not unusual reactions to this unsettling experience. After some thirty-odd years of fairly regular and familiar menstruation, with the occasional variations a woman has grown to recognize, a woman now enters a period of unexpected and unfamiliar bleeding. Sometimes there is too much, at other times too little. Sometimes it is too soon, sometimes too late. Is she pregnant? Is the bleeding a menstrual period or hemorrhaging? Is the blood a sign of cancer? Is there blood because of last night's or yesterday's sex?

The hurried frantic call to the doctor is not to be dismissed as the neurotic fears of middle-aged ladies. Consultation with the physician about these changed patterns of menstruation, to rule out causes other than normal menopause, makes far better sense than ignoring what might be warning signals of a potentially serious condition. Regular expert medical checkups are in order to assure both the patient and the physician that the irregularity is part of the normal sequence of events—in most women this is the case.

Many women, when they first experience a missed period as a result of their waning reproductive years, express surprise and even denial that it could be happening to them. One can look young and be vigorous, with as many years ahead to live as were lived while reproduction was possible, and yet be at the aging end of reproductive ability. A frequent response is the surprise or concern at the possibility that the missed period is a sign of pregnancy. And sometimes this brush with the possibility of pregnancy brings women into close confrontation with other aspects of their lives. Several women have described their reactions:

> The first time my period was two weeks late was when I was close to forty. It never occurred to me that it might be a sign of menopause—I felt and looked young. I was sure I was pregnant. It almost ruined my marriage. I hadn't planned a baby, but the idea of having another child was a sort of nice surprise. My husband was hysterical. He called from work every day—Did I call the doctor to see if I needed an abortion. I began to wonder if he loved me.

Another woman said:

> In my mid-forties, for the first time, I began to have an affair. I had never enjoyed sex as much as with my lover. Then one month I skipped my period. I was really frightened. When it finally came, I was so grateful I swore I would never get involved with a man other than my husband.

Some women deny that they are experiencing the symptomatology of menopause. One woman I know never missed an opportunity to announce, "I have my period. I'm menstruating like a sixteen-year-old." The following woman had a positive experience:

> When I was in my mid-forties I began to have very irregular periods. Sometimes they were late, sometimes they were early. Sometimes the flow was heavy, sometimes, light. It was kind of nerve wracking. I was lucky. I went to a gynecologist who gave me a very thorough examination. He assured me that my body was healthy and that there were no pathological conditions. I returned for semi-annual checkups. Over the next few years my periods gradually became less frequent and when I was fifty-three I had my last one. I am grateful for the reassurance of that doctor, and I'm glad that he didn't push estrogen.

The final ending of the menstrual period or, in the quaint term of the older medical writers, "the retention of the menses," does of course *not* mean that a woman need no longer continue with medical checkups. On the contrary, since increasing age is associated with increased susceptibility to various ills, good medical care remains essential.

## The Physiology of Menopause and Menstruation

The disturbances in menstrual flow that come around the time of menopause are the result of changes in the lining of the uterus, which are themselves the result of changes in the hormonal balance of the body. These changing conditions are perhaps best understood in relation to the conditions in the human female body that precede menopause.

Almost as if in a grand burst of optimism, or perhaps simply in order to take no chances that humanity might not reproduce itself, the female infant is provided with some 40,000 to 300,000 follicles or cells containing immature eggs. These follicles are contained in the almond-shaped glands, the ovaries, which are a major component of the female genital system. Over the course of the reproductive years, each month one of these follicles, occasionally more than one, will mature, its maturing egg will be released upon the rupturing of the follicle. This release of the mature ovum generally takes place during the fourteenth to twenty-fifth day of the menstrual cycle. The egg then moves down the fallopian tubes to the uterus. It is here that the egg can be fertilized by male sperm. If one egg is released—the most usual situation—and fertilized by male sperm, the result will be one human embryo, although should that fertilized egg divide into two, fraternal twins can result. If more than one egg is released, twins, triplets, etc., can result, depending on the number of ovum released and fertilized. Most women bear single babies, although twins are also not uncommon. But, until the recent use of fertility drugs stimulated more than one ovarian follicle to rupture, multiple births of four, five, and six children were extremely rare. Occasionally an ovum is fertilized in the fallopian tubes and remains there. This type of pregnancy, called ectopic pregnancy, presents a danger to the mother because the fallopian tubes cannot contain a growing embryo without rupturing. An ectopic pregnancy requires surgical intervention—the pain and bleeding associated with it, fortunately, make the patient seek medical attention promptly.

If the ovum is not fertilized, it merely disintegrates and is discharged.

The ovarian follicle has another function to perform besides that of producing the ripening egg, and that is the function of preparing estrogen and progesterone which, among other things, prepare the lining of the womb for the nourishment and protection of a fertilized ovum. Without this preparation, which includes the thickening of the lining of the womb (the endometrium) and the formation of glands, and the increase of blood supply in the endometrium, a fertilized egg could not implant itself in the womb, the fertilized egg would be discharged, and pregnancy made impossible.

During the first half of the menstrual cycle (five to fourteen days after the onset of menstruation) estrogen causes the uterine lining to grow. The ovum is then released and begins its journey through the fallopian tubes to the womb—a journey that may take about six and one-half days. During this time after the rupture of the ovarian follicle, the secretion of the hormone progesterone further prepares the lining of the womb for the reception of a fertilized egg.

Menstruation is the shedding of the uterine lining, which occurs when there is no pregnancy. It occurs because the level of estrogen and progesterone drop. The entire cycle of follicle maturation, estrogen production, follicle rupture, progesterone production, and ovum journey, to shedding of the endometrium, takes about twenty-eight days, the familiar monthly period. The actual number of days can vary. It can vary from month to month in the same woman, and its duration can differ among women.

The cycle continues to repeat itself throughout the reproductive life span of a woman, although at the beginning years and the last years of menstruation there is likely to be irregularity and decreased chances of pregnancy due to changing hormonal conditions. The action of the ovaries in producing hormones is not independent. The ovaries are themselves influenced by the follicle-stimulating hormone (FSH) secreted by the pituitary gland—the "master" gland situated at the base of the skull. The complex and sensitive interrelationships within the endocrine gland system of the body are demonstrated by the fact that on about the fifth day of the menstrual cycle (the fifth day after the onset of menstruation) the low level of estrogen seems to trigger the pituitary gland to send out the hormones to stimulate the ovary to begin producing another mature ovum.

The actions of the contraceptive pills are based upon this intricate balance between the hormones in the body. The pill contains estrogen, which keeps the level in the body high enough to keep the pituitary gland from sending out FSH to start the maturation of an ovum. Therefore, no egg is produced. With no egg there can be no pregnancy. Pretty much the same thing happens during pregnancy. The pregnant woman has a high enough level of estrogen to inhibit the pituitary from acting on the ovarian follicles, and in this way no further pregnancy can occur until after she has given birth. The contraceptive pill contains a combination of estrogen and progesterone to enable the shedding of the uterine lining to take place on schedule each month, unlike the condition of actual pregnancy.

Somewhere, for most women between the ages of forty-five and fifty-five, changing hormonal balance leads to the ending of the menstrual cycle—the menopause. For the majority of women, the change is gradual and without difficulties. For a minority, the imbalance resulting from the physiological changes in the endocrine gland system may require medical attention. It is estimated, in the United States, that about 25 per cent of women of menopausal age go to their doctors precisely because of "menopausal" symptoms. It cannot be presumed that all others have no symptoms, of course, since many women simply ignore or endure, as the case may be, manifestation of their menopause. Nor can it be assumed that the symptoms are necessarily caused by menopause. It can be expected that what is considered normal at some times can become cause for medical treatment according to current fashion and belief. For example, with the recent expansion of introducing estrogen for women at menopause, ordinary normal menstrual irregularity was treated as requiring medication. Also, the "hot flush" was depicted in the ads of the drug manufacturers as well as in advice given women by their favorite magazines, as a totally unnecessary condition. Many women who otherwise might have justifiably ignored their flushes, especially when relatively mild, were now, because of fashion, more likely to seek medical intervention.

Menstrual irregularities can be traced to the fact that toward the end of the reproductive cycle, as a woman nears menopause, there is usually a decline in the amount of estrogen which is produced by the ovarian follicles, as well as a decline in the estrogen-progesterone secretion of the corpus luteum (a hormone-secreting gland formed in the ovary). Skipped or delayed menstrual periods result from a follicle having matured late. Sometimes a scanty flow is the result of lessened material in the lining of the womb, even though an ovum may have matured. The pituitary gland continues to produce its hormones, but there is a gradual decline in ovulation as well as appropriate preparation of the womb, thus lessening, but not completely eradicating, the possibility of conception and pregnancy.

By the time a woman reaches her middle years she is very familiar with the characteristics of her menstruation and regards that bleeding as regular. With the irregularity that comes with the menopause years, there is the understandable concern that the vaginal discharge might possibly be abnormal and, at the very worst, a sign of cancer. Most women do not get cancer. It is true, however, that the incidence of cancer of the cervix is highest at about age forty-nine in the United States, and the rate of cancer of the endometrium (lining of the womb) is at its highest about the age of fifty-nine. Because of this, it is essential that women have pelvic examinations regularly, and that these include a Papanicolaou smear—popularly known as the Pap test—of the cervix and endocervix which can indicate the presence of cancer or precancerous conditions of the cervix. If taken ten days after a menstrual period the smear can also indicate pathology of the lining of the womb. In some women, excessive frequency or amount of bleeding, or grossly irregular bleeding might require a surgical curettage, scraping of the lining of the womb; a safe and rapid procedure when done under modern hospital conditions.

For the majority of women, menopause is uneventful. For those who at this time of their lives happen to be ill, early diagnosis is the wisest course.

The physiological change from the ability to reproduce to a post-reproductive stage of a woman's life does not happen suddenly. The so-called "climacteric," the term for this change, may take several years. Indeed, some change is always occurring in the human female. Born with the extravagant number of ovarian follicles, the processes leading to development and aging go on through life, the body apparently in a state of exquisite synchronization. It is sobering to keep in mind that evidence of pubertal changes can be observed in girls well before menarche (first menstruation), and menarche itself can appear before the actual ability to reproduce; and the endocrinological changes preceding menopause also appear gradually until the balance is tipped in favor of menopause. The event of first menstruation, frequently celebrated in ritual by people around the

world is particularly dramatic as a symbol of change to a reproductive status. Actually, however, in some cases conception can precede menstruation—among the Ibo of Nigeria, children born of such
conceptions were regarded as abominations. And, as noted above,
menstruation by itself does not insure simultaneous fertility—sometimes a period of sterility of several months or longer may follow the
first menstruation.

The event of menopause is hardly as dramatic as menarche. Its
symptomology can precede the actual end of menstruation because
the shifts in hormonal balance are unlikely to occur suddenly; and,
until at least a year has passed since the last menstruation, there is
also the possibility that a mature ovum can be fertilized and im-
planted in a receptive womb.

In this age of expanded knowledge concerning the endocrine system of the body, as well as sophisticated laboratory techniques, there
are other ways of determining whether or not a woman's menstrual
irregularities or other symptoms are a function of menopause. This
involves the analysis of vaginal smears and urine. However, these
techniques are not always reliable. In the case of the vaginal smear, it
is possible to determine the estrogen level, and the absence or
marked decrease in estrogen is indicative of the end of ovarian function. But there are some problems with this method of analysis.[2] For
one thing, even ordinarily the level of estrogen is variable from day
to day. For another, it is now known that the ending of menstruation does not mean that the ovaries stop secreting estrogen. Some
function continues, and there is evidence that the majority of
women continue to show estrogenic vaginal smears for ten years after
menopause. Severe atrophy, that is, absence of estrogen, is found in
only 25 per cent of women within a ten-year period after menopause.
Vaginal smears are also subject to alteration by the presence of other
hormones, medications, or local infections, and these can produce
misleading results. Urinary estrogen secretion is also present, indicating estrogen production.

It appears that some ovarian function continues, and it is believed
that the adrenal glands take over some of the function of producing
estrogen, the source of urinary estrogen. One urine test determines
whether or not there is an increase in the amount of pituitary gona-
dotrophin secretion (follicle stimulating hormone). Apparently, in
an effort to stimulate the lagging ovaries the pituitary gland produces

more of this hormone at menopause, and this can be detected in the urine.

These techniques for determining the hormonal conditions that characterize menopause are useful to the physician in regard to diagnosis of menopause, or diagnosis of severe hormonal imbalance. What is perhaps most interesting is that on the basis of these sophisticated techniques, it is now known that most women at menopause do not enter into a state of severe estrogen deprivation. Estrogen production continues, although at a lower level, as the body seeks to establish a new balance, or homeostasis.

Despite their limitations, laboratory techniques for diagnosis of the menopause are invaluable diagnostic aids to the physician when he is confronted with the need to determine whether a patient is indicating menopausal symptoms or whether there are other, potentially serious reasons for the symptoms. For example, the absence of menstruation can be the result of a serious condition such as hypothyroidism; the "hot flush" of menopause is mimicked by the night diaphoresis (sweats) of some chronic infections such as tuberculosis. The careful physician will rule out these possibilities in questionable cases.

## Hot Flushes

Another of the classic symptoms of menopause has been described widely as "hot flush." Sometimes called flashes or sweats, these are vasomotor symptoms, which are as yet imperfectly understood by the medical community. Not all women experience this vasomotor instability, and of those who do, most experience a mild variety—only occasional and very transitory periods of warmth, lasting a few seconds or minutes.

Hot flushes have been described as a wave of heat spreading over the upper half of the body to the face, sometimes accompanied by sweating and followed by a chill. Since sweating cools the body, a feeling of coolness or chill is not strange following the experience of heat. The on-again-off-again tossing of the bed covers at night, the opening of windows in rooms where others are cool, the tampering with the thermostat, and search for sleeveless dresses in the cold winter have become grist for the mill of comedians' and men's jokes, often in very bad taste. For most women, again, the hot flush is either not experienced or, when it is, it is no more than a mild, often unnoticed sensation. For others the hot flush is an acutely uncomfortable experience, including profuse and embarrassing, sometimes frightening, sweats requiring changes of bed linens at night, and clothes during the day. A hot flush can last anywhere from one half a minute to three minutes. They can occur up to ten to twelve times a day.

Hot flushes, when they do occur, appear at the end of the menopause and are usually a postmenopausal symptom.

Why do some women have them more than others? Despite the apparent universality of the symptom—although some peoples like Gypsies and the women of the Caucasus do not complain of hot flushes[3]—the physiology is still not well understood, although it is known to be related to a disturbance or imbalance of the autonomic nervous system. It may be due to an estrogen deficiency—estrogen is believed to protect the subcutaneous blood vessels—and until the body re-establishes an internal balance, or homeostasis, the vasomotor symptom persists. It is known that women undergoing sudden artificial menopause due to hysterectomy experience flushes. It is also known that estrogen administration relieves the symptoms.

The hot flush may also have a psychosomatic component. There is an element of self-fulfilling prophecy about it since many women expect to experience hot flushes. There is also the matter of how a woman perceives her experience with flushes compared with others. The analogy most women will recognize is that of attitude toward menstruation. A minor discomfort to one girl was the justification for staying home from school or skipping gym class; for another, the same degree of discomfort was ignored as participation in both classes and athletics continued. This is not to deny that some women do have a more uncomfortable flush, but the fact is that some women are more tolerant of variations in their body sensations than are others. Some women are also unnecessarily frightened by their experience—hot flushes can't harm you—and become anxious, only to have their symptoms grow worse.

There is, in addition, a cultural component to "hot flushes." Contrary to what might be expected, not all women in the world want to do without hot flushes, nor do they care to relieve their intensity. Among the women of a South Wales mining town, for example, hot flushes are believed to be good for you—the more frequent the better! in order to insure that dangerous complications will not occur.[4]

They believed that flushes were caused by menstrual blood rushing to the head, so that an absence of flushes meant a dangerous deficiency of menstrual blood. In this region there is a popular saying: "A flush is worth a guinea a box" (a reference to a pre-World War II laxative advertisement) because flushes are believed to carry one safely and quickly through the menopause. Among these women, to *not* have hot flushes is something they are somewhat embarrassed about and will sometimes apologize that they are "not very good at it."

For some native village women in Jamaica the experience of the hot flush is explained in terms of witchcraft or spirit possession. For example, in one case a woman said she was "feeling heat like somebody had fire to her tail." She believed others saw the fire—the heat was so hot she felt it had to be fire. She would then exclaim: "You see it! You see the fire!" The woman believed that "duppy" or "spirits" were causing her trouble, and for relief went to the Obeah man (medicine man). For treatment he prescribed that she boil nine different bushes and bathe in the water for nine mornings. After that, she should get a calabash (a local gourd), mix the guts with castor oil and drink the mixture; this would clean out her body and bring back her health, and the sweating and heat would disappear.[5]

Another Jamaican woman treated her hot flush symptom by collecting Cerase—a vine with small leaves, used as a cure for many things including skin diseases and internal complaints—and boiling it, using it as a tea and instead of water when she felt thirsty. Her husband bought an earthenware pot, and bottled the Cerase using the wine as a preservative. The woman drank a wine glass full twice a day as a tonic. One is reminded of the old Lydia Pinkham home remedy for all female complaints so popular in the United States in the last century—probably due to its alcohol base. At any rate, whether from the Cerase, the wine, or time, the flashes and the sweats lessened in severity.

It is difficult to tell whether or not the herbal baths or tea of the Jamaican were effective relief of hot flushes over and beyond any mere placebo effect. We are certain that menstrual blood rushing to the head, as believed by the Welsh women, is not the physical cause of the symptom, although the sense of loss of menstruation might induce some women to treasure their menses—what we do not know is that the prescription for the relief of symptoms given by modern Western doctors, the estrogen drugs which were so eagerly grasped by despairing women impatient with their discomfort, was hardly the wisest of medications. Now that the dangers of administration of the drug have become known, physician and patient must weigh extremely carefully the use of estrogen therapy to relieve hot flushes. Indeed, some women have now found that they can more easily bear their discomfort than expose themselves to risk. One would hope that the medical community would increase its research efforts in this area, better to understand the nature of the vasomotor disturbances experienced by women and, hopefully, to find a remedy or remedies that are simple and effective.

Irregularity of the menstrual cycle and hot flushes are symptoms that ovarian function is changing. Most women do not consult their doctors about menopausal symptoms because they are either absent or not so severe or disturbing to make them do so. Other women, either because they routinely seek medical assistance, or because of anxiety over possible pregnancy or unfamiliar symptoms, do.

Good medical care is advisable to reassure women that their symptoms are normal reactions to normal changes in body functioning and chemistry. However, a very real problem can arise if many of the possible real complaints a woman may have are casually dismissed because of her age as "menopausal." For example, there is a whole list of ailments common to middle-aged women—and middle-aged men and others as well—that have been carelessly lumped together as "menopausal syndrome." These include backache, headache, vertigo (dizziness), fatigue—that terrible tired feeling—irritability, tingling sensations, weight increase, and forgetfulness. Women complaining of these and assorted other aches and pains deserve as careful a medical diagnosis as any man or woman of another age presenting these symptoms. In recent years the ads of the estrogen manufacturers directed at the medical community have urged the use of hormones to treat these complaints and have built up a picture, vividly displayed in multicolored, multipaged, glossy ads of the distressed, nervous, cranky, uncomfortable, middle-aged lady whose complaints can be traced to "menopausal syndrome." One such nasty ad tells doctors to give hormones "when your patient has outlived her ovaries."

Is there any truth in this combination of ills that can be traced to menopause? Or are these symptoms of other problems? Is it just fashionable in our time and culture to associate these with menopause, or are they really a related set of difficulties?

# Menopause — Is It Necessary?

## THE SEARCH FOR IMMORTALITY AND THE ESTROGEN CONTROVERSY

Is menopause a necessary condition for the mature human female? Is it part of a natural design of growth, development, and decline which carries each human being from conception through birth, maturity, and death? Or is it some biological accident that should not really occur, now that the life expectancy of women has reached a point where, for many, the postmenopausal years are as long as the childbearing years? Is menopause a disease, a pathology, with symptoms responding to diagnosis and treatment for prevention and cure?

These are not frivolous questions, for how one regards the phenomenon of menopause is fundamental to how it is accepted or treated, as the case may be. They involve significant differences in philosophy of analysis and medical care.

If it is believed that there is a "wisdom of the body" by which delicate hormonal balance is achieved naturally, the body resisting attempts to interfere, then medical intervention is minimal. On the other hand, the large-scale routine administration of the hormone estrogen to so many menopausal and postmenopausal women in the 1960s and early 1970s stems from a belief that the body is deficient, ill, out of balance, and requires help.

All women who survive through their forties and fifties experience menopause, with the very rare exception of a very late menstruating woman. It used to be argued that the human female was the only female in all the animal kingdom to experience the end of reproductive function as she is the only female to be continuously able to engage in sexual activity. Among the primate species, who are closest to mankind, the females do not menstruate regularly, but rather have an oestrus cycle, a period of receptivity to sexual activity during which they are able to conceive, and which is evidenced by swelling and coloration of their genitalia. Human menstruation and the oestrus cycle are not identical—humans ordinarily do not conceive during menstruation and receptivity depends more on the place, the time, and the partner and does not end even when reproduction is no longer possible. Still, the absence of an end to oestrus cycles seemed to mock the human condition, to suggest that there was something wrong with menopause since it was not seen in our primate relatives.

But there is new evidence that even among the monkeys, reproductive ability on the part of the female does not go on forever. Now that monkeys, for example, have been in captivity over a long period of time, older females are seen without the oestrus cycle: not exactly menopause, but an indication that long life brings changes in reproductive cycles to primate females other than humans.

The answer to the question of why menopause occurs is much more difficult to answer than the question of how it occurs.

With similar patterns of development observable among humans and primates, there is support for the notion that menopause is indeed a normal condition, that it is part of the natural developmental pattern of growth and physiology experienced in the life of the female of the species. In support of this point of view one leading gynecologist has written, "The menopause can perhaps be regarded as a physiological phenomenon which is protective in nature—protective from undesirable reproduction and the associated growth stimuli."[1]

Menopause seen as a protective device is one way of handling the question of why it occurs. But the answer is still uncertain. Although some women survived into late years throughout history, it is only in very modern times that the average age of life—and, at that, only in the advanced industrial countries—is well above the age of menopause. With the average of menopause around the age of fifty, and the average life expectancy for women going above seventy, almost one third of a woman's life in modern nations is now lived after menopause. Was it because people died at earlier ages that a design for continuing reproductive capacity was not important? The evolutionary course of menopause is one that defies definitive answers given the present state of knowledge. Whatever the reason, again, all human females experience the shift in endocrine hormone balance, which leads to the end of reproductive capacity and the end of menstruation.

The analysis of menopause as a natural physiological development characteristic of the human species leads to an attitude of acceptance, a medical program of support over any unusual difficulties experienced by a minority of women, and as little tampering with the natural process of the body as possible as it makes continuing adjustments to changing phases of the life cycle.

But mankind has never been about to settle for the world as he finds it and inevitably seeks to improve upon it. And menopause especially lends itself to efforts to make it disappear. This is particularly true in societies where menopause is a stigmatizing event associated with the loss of the ability to bear children and believed to cause the loss of youth and beauty.

The search for a way to forestall the process of aging is not limited to women. Ponce de León was on a male quest for the fountain of youth. For women the answer seemed to have come from a whole other direction. If ovarian failure and the subsequent decline in production of the hormones estrogen and progesterone was the how of menopause, the answer to the problem of retaining everlasting youth seemed to be found in the replacement of those hormones by the modern miracles of chemistry.

This cultural attitude supports the very valid scientific question concerning whether or not menopause is an illness, as yet imperfectly understood, a condition to be treated somewhat the way in which diabetes is treated. And, if menopause is an illness, what are its symptoms? Lumped together are a set of signs that are supposed to characterize menopause. These are vasomotor complaints such as flushes, sweats, palpitations, muscle cramps, and faintness, and a whole host of emotional complaints in addition: depression, nervousness, anxiety, restless nights, fatigue.

As far as treatment is concerned, in diabetes the pancreas does not produce insulin, therefore the patient is given insulin—the illness treated but not cured. In menopause, the ovary does not produce adequate estrogen, therefore supporters of this viewpoint urged the need to give the patient exogenous (from the outside) estrogen.

One of the foremost advocates of this position was Dr. Robert Wilson, author of the book *Feminine Forever*, a widely read and influential book of the early 1960s.[2] What a seductive theory! And what a seductive title to entice women and their doctors to begin using, routinely, the new estrogen preparations throughout their lives, to replace the hormones their bodies were supposedly no longer producing. Estrogen hormones had been on the market for some twenty years previous, but they were now being plugged for use in what became known as estrogen replacement therapy—or, as one of the leading drug manufacturers urged, "Keep Her on Premarin" (a leading estrogen product) or to give "when a woman outlives her ovaries."

Now, there is a significant difference between the use of estrogens by physicians on a short-term or intermittent basis for the amelioration of certain occasional serious difficulties experienced by individual women. But the advocates of routine hormone replacement for a whole generation of women were arguing that menopause is a deficiency disease, and that the most dreadful things would happen to all women if they didn't get estrogen. They implied that femininity was about to be lost, bones would disintegrate, skin would collapse in wrinkled folds, sexual organs would shrink or grow. One writer even spoke of the growing size of the clitoris, as if without estrogen women were about to develop penises, which does not happen.[3] They talked about growth of body hair and various other horrors that implied women were about to turn into castrates, devoid of their sexuality, even their appearance as women. They wrote as if women in their forties—a glorious time of life when many women are more vigorous and beautiful than ever—were about to turn into aged crones, as if reaching menopause was like leaving Shangri La—with youth and beauty vanishing without a trace.

This dangerous nonsense was unfortunately popularized by Dr. David Reuben, writing in the popular, *Everything You Always Wanted to Know about Sex but Were Afraid to Ask:*

> As the estrogen is shut off, a woman comes as close as she can to becoming a man, increased facial hair, deepened voice, obesity, and the decline of the breasts and female genitalia all contribute to a masculine appearance. Coarsened features, enlargement of the clitoris, a gradual baldness complete the tragic picture. Not really a man but no longer a woman, these individuals live in the world of intersex.[4]

While this sounds more like a medical textbook description of the extremely rare androgen syndrome, it also echoed the multimillion-dollar drug industry's campaign to sell estrogen. The phenomenal growth in sales led to a point where five million prescriptions of estrogen drugs were sold in the United States in 1974 while only some one and one-half million women were actually in the menopausal years. The high prescription rate is attributable to the increasing numbers of postmenopausal women on these drugs in a routine program of estrogen replacement.

In addition to "educational" campaigns by the drug manufacturers among doctors was the great publicity given estrogen replacement by the leading women's magazines. They ran features on looking fabulous after forty, feeling great over forty, good news about menopause, with articles implying everlasting loveliness with estrogen thrown in. In general, their advice on grooming, diet, and exercise was exemplary and indeed an asset to the woman wishing to keep her attractiveness, but the advice on estrogen was unfortunate. One of the leading writers for these magazines was psychiatrist Dr. M. Dorothea Kerr, an advocate of estrogen therapy.[5] One article by Dr. Kerr advocating estrogen replacement therapy, issued as a very elegantly printed brochure, complete with photographs and lists of menopausal complaints, was distributed widely by the Ayerst Corporation, manufacturer of Premarin. The brochure included a full-page description of the drug. However, although including a reference to full product information on the package, the brochure conveniently left out the long list of contraindications for the drug use.[6]

The Ayerst laboratories also maintained an "Information Center for the Mature Woman," located in New York, and distributed widely information on menopause advocating estrogen replacement therapy for the so-called "menopausal syndrome." When the Food and Drug Administration, in 1976, called attention to the increased rates of cancer of the uterus that were beginning to be apparent, the Information Center closed its operation. It would seem that had their primary function been informational rather than that of advocating the use of the drug, they would have had more work than ever to do and more information to dispense. Instead, they simply closed down.

## Estrogens and Cancer

Women who had routinely been using estrogen replacement therapy for its supposedly beneficial effects in preventing the negative aspects of menopause—either because they had been led to believe that menopause was an unnecessary "disease," or because of severe symptoms which required alleviation—received a rude shock with the publication of evidence that estrogen replacement was linked with cancer of the womb. The illusive quest for perpetual youth met still another impasse with the steadily mounting evidence that taking estrogen—the hormone that promised a miraculous passage through the middle and later years—for long periods of time caused cancer. Like Dr. Steinbach's transplantation of the glands of the ram and the sheep to the human body for the purposes of rejuvenation, a century ago, or the monkey gland advocate of the early twentieth century, another effort to defer the effects of time clashed head on with the human body, moving on its own inexorable way through life.

A major study, published in the prestigious *New England Journal of Medicine* in 1976, carefully documented the conclusion that there is a clear relationship between exogenous estrogen (estrogen taken into the body from outside in the form of drugs, as opposed to estrogen normally produced by the body) and the rising incidence of endometrial cancer in the United States (cancer of the lining of the uterus, the major source of cancer of the body of the uterus).[7]

In this study, Dr. Noel S. Weiss and his colleagues, working at the University of Washington, the Fred Hutchinson Cancer Research Center, and the State of California Department of Health, point to the rapid increase in incidence of endometrial cancer of a magnitude that has rarely been paralleled in the history of cancer reporting in this country—an increase of 10 per cent per year in some areas during the 1970s. The incidence among middle-aged women has changed most, by 40 to 150 per cent between 1969 and 1973, depending on the area, but rates have changed among younger women and older women as well. It seems highly unlikely that this magnitude of increase reported throughout the United States can be accounted for simply by new methods of diagnosing and reporting.

The evidence for the relationship between the use of estrogen preparations by menopausal women as being at the very least in part responsible for this rise in incidence of cancer is based on three types of evidence. One is evidence on the association of estrogen produced by the body with cancer, the second is the frequency of use of exogenous estrogen among women with this form of cancer, and the third is the time relationship between the period of increased estrogen consumption and the present rise in incidence of the disease.

It has been known for some time that increased estrogen levels over the normal appear to predispose women to endometrial cancer. This has been shown among women with estrogen-secreting ovarian tumors and in young women given prolonged treatment with stilbes-trol (a chemical estrogen).

The evidence kept mounting that women on exogenous estrogens seemed to have as much as a seven times greater risk of endometrial cancer compared with non-users.

But for menopausal women the evidence was far less clear. After all, with estrogen levels declining it did not seem so strange to keep the levels up. Besides, estrogen for menopausal women has been prescribed for only the last several years compared with the thirty-year history of estrogen use in general, so there was little experience with the long-term effects of estrogen when given to women in the menopausal years. The phenomenal growth in estrogen use now posed new problems.

The United States Department of Commerce reports, for example, that there has been a steady, rapid increase in the amount of non-contraceptive shipments of estrogen within the United States for human consumption during the past decade. The value of these drugs in 1973 was nearly $70,000,000 and by 1976, $80,000,000. In one survey of the Seattle-Tacoma area, it was estimated that 51 per cent of menopausal women in these communities had used "replace-ment" estrogens for at least three months, and that the median dura-tion of use was ten years. It seems that it was the women experienc-ing menopause in the late 1960s and the 1970s who were most exposed. Many of these were women in high socioeconomic brackets with the best medical care, receiving the very latest in fashionable medicine, and responding to the advice of the leading women's mag-azines of the country that they could stay youthful and fantastic for-ever by taking these miracle drugs. The multimillion-dollar drug in-dustry with its glossy advertising copy graced medical journals throughout the world contrasting a distraught, gray-haired woman with a radiant-looking, attractive woman, advising physicians to "Put Her on Premarin" and "Keep Her There."

Despite its promise of well-being, estrogen, like all other drugs, has contraindications or conditions under which it should not be admin-istered because of the dangers it might pose to the person taking it. In the case of estrogen, the contraindications are many—although the glossy ads for the drugs relegate the contraindications to the fine print, sometimes not even on the same page as the fancy blurbs ex-tolling the virtues of the drug. Women with small leiomyomas (benign tumors) of the uterus require special care in relation to estrogen. Some believe that hormone therapy, when necessary, can be started but the woman receiving hormones under these conditions must be examined frequently. Should the tumors increase in size, the drug must not be taken. Since some 50 per cent of women over forty have small fibroid tumors, this means that millions of women are at risk.

Breast cancer is another contraindication to estrogen use. So is migraine headache; women with this condition also must be careful for should the headaches increase in severity or frequency then hormone treatment should be suspended.

Any history of heart difficulty is also a problem. This is the probable reason: all estrogen preparations act in such a way so that salt (sodium) is retained by the body—the common reason why women on birth-control pills frequently complain about swelling. For those women with a medical history of edema, or swelling, or women who have a history of heart or circulatory difficulty, estrogen is contraindicated and should not be administered. And, as if the above were not enough reasons not to administer estrogen, anyone with a case history of kidney or liver disease also cannot take estrogen for that hormone is metabolized in the liver and excreted in the urine.

Even perfectly healthy women taking the drug were subject to adverse reactions. These included: nausea, vomiting, anorexia (loss of appetite), gastrointestinal symptoms such as abdominal cramps and bloating, breakthrough bleeding (non-menstrual), spotting, unusually heavy withdrawal bleeding, breast tenderness and enlargement, reactivation of endometriosis (spread of endometrial tissue), possible lowered milk production when given to mothers after childbirth, edema, aggravation of migraine headaches, change in body weight (either an increase or a decrease), allergic rash, and/or hepatic cutaneous porphyria (abdominal pain and nervousness) becoming manifest.

Despite this long list of when one must not take estrogen, or what it might most unhappily do, many women, unaware of the dangers, swore by the beneficial results of the drug—their purported sense of well-being, the belief that they looked and felt better, the relief of some of the unwelcome symptoms of menopause such as a severe hot flush, making them receptive to use of the drug.

As exogenous estrogen began to be used with some regularity as replacement therapy amongst postmenopausal women, so did evidence begin to mount that this routine administration of drugs presented real dangers, aside from cancer.

In one study, undertaken in Boston by the Boston Collaborative Drug Surveillance Program, over five thousand postmenopausal women aged forty-five to sixty were monitored to determine the effect of estrogen-containing drugs. This particular survey found no significant association between the use of estrogen and such conditions as venous thromboembolism (blood clots in the veins) or breast tumors. However, it did find a highly significant increase in the incidence of surgically confirmed gall-bladder disease in women who took estrogen as compared with a group of women who did not. The risk of developing gall-bladder disease was increased two and one-half times among the women on estrogen.[8]

It was estimated that the incidence rate of gall-bladder disease presumably attributable to estrogen use was 131 cases per 100,-000,000 women. While this leaves the overwhelming majority of women on estrogen replacement therapy free from the possibility of contracting this illness, it nonetheless points to the dangers presented to some—and the risk every woman took when on this regimen.

Now that large numbers of menopausal women have been exposed to exogenous estrogens, the paralleling rise in the rate of endometrial cancer supports the other evidence indicating a causal link.

In another major study of endometrial cancer, this time among the women of an affluent retirement community, Dr. Thomas Mack and his associates found evidence that supports at a high level of statistical significance, the hypothesis that exogenous estrogens cause endometrial cancer.[9]

What should a woman do when told she needs estrogen replacement therapy in the face of this disastrous news concerning uterine cancer?

For one thing, as Dr. Mack and his colleagues point out, estrogen is not something like smoking cigarettes, which we know to be dangerous, but which somehow you can manage to continue doing optionally. Rather, estrogen is like those valuable but potentially dangerous drugs such as insulin and digitalis. Insulin is useful to prevent the greater danger of diabetic coma, and the potent drug digitalis enables the faltering heart to continue functioning. Estrogen is useful only when serious medical conditions warrant it. And *when pre-scribed, it should be at the minimal dosage and over the shortest possible time.* To use estrogen for the relief of an occasional hot flush or in the hopes it will preserve one's youth is courting disaster—you don't die from hot flushes or wrinkles. To trade a minor ailment for a possibly lethal cure is scarcely the sensible course. And millions of American women are now shunning the use of estrogen at menopause.

With the recent exposé it is likely that estrogen prescriptions will no longer be casually offered to menopausal women. The medical community itself has become increasingly concerned, and the United States Food and Drug Administration has been advised to limit strictly the use of estrogen for the symptoms and aftereffects of menopause.[10] It looks as if the idea that a woman should be on estrogen replacement therapy routinely until she dies is out. Although the current $80,000,000 market for estrogen may or may not suffer a severe depression as a result, it is likely that American physicians, at least, are likely to be very cautious concerning this routine—regular estrogen replacement—given the fear of malpractice suits should endometrial cancer appear in the patient.

Estrogen is no different from any other drug in that it should be taken only for a therapeutic reason—if a woman is ill, or extremely uncomfortable and a medical cure is available, then she has the right to seek it. But the informed woman will have to weigh, together with an informed physician, the pros and cons of treatment, how sick she is, and the alternative forms of treatment against the potential action of the drug. Occasional menstrual irregularity, an occasional hot flush or night sweat, or a "tired" feeling that may have to do more with some dissatisfaction with one's life—difficult children, an exhausting job, widowhood, a roving husband, the sense of now or never in terms of one's own fulfillment, or an elusive search for warding off the inevitable years—do not seem to warrant unnecessary exposure to the effects of estrogen replacement. A forthright confrontation with the realities of life and a thorough physical examination to rule out real physical disability unrelated to menopause to reassure one of fitness seem far more realistic. A woman's physical complaints deserve careful attention. To simply dismiss them as "menopausal" is unwarranted. In the absence of especially serious symptoms, estrogen should not be taken casually.

Unfortunately, now that the use of estrogen is likely to be far more restricted, and informed women far less likely to expose themselves to risk, the dangers of increased incidence of uterine disease are not yet over. Some five million prescriptions for estrogen were written in 1974 alone. The effects of these drugs are not likely to be seen for a period of from four to eight years, since the effects are generally delayed.

Since women over forty have been using estrogens over the past several years, they are justifiably concerned about their individual states of health now that the evidence is in. Fortunately, however, the statistical chances for becoming ill are still relatively slim for the individual. Having been on estrogen does not necessarily mean that cancer of the womb will develop.

## Is There a Menopausal Syndrome?

Estrogen may not be the answer, but is there a "menopausal syndrome" which *does* require medical attention?

There remains a dearth of really solid research on the physiology of older women. K. J. Lennane and R. J. Lennane, writing in the *New England Journal of Medicine* as recently as 1973, point out that sexism applies in regard to the alleged psychogenic (biologically related) disorders in women.[11] While medical research and evidence is relatively plentiful in relation to the disorders of younger women, there is an astonishingly small amount of attention paid to the older woman, with traditional attitudes holding sway over the absence of careful research. In the absence of the careful investigations concerning the biological relationship of menopause, or the climacteric, upon the psychological disorders and other physical manifestations observed among women of that age, it remains impossible to definitively answer the question concerning whether or not women have problems at menopause because of their biology. But there remains an enormous amount of evidence from around the world that how women react to and experience menopause, except perhaps for the two universal symptoms of no longer menstruating experienced by all and the hot flush and night sweat experienced by some, depends on the social conditions of life experienced by women as they move from the status of procreative women to the stage of life beyond.

Women have a right to ask why there has been such minimal

medical attention to a major event in the life of every woman who survives through middle age compared with the attention given younger women. In part, this reflects the double standard accorded older women vs. younger women in our society. The menopause, in Western cultures, as pointed out by Sonja M. McKinlay and John B. McKinlay of the Harvard University Medical School and Department of Sociology, Cambridge, is a ". . . stigmatizing event in a woman's life marking the end of her social usefulness—procreation. This attitude has been perpetuated in the cursory consideration given by the medical profession to the relief of any accompanying uncomfortable symptoms—an attitude clearly reflected in even recent gynecology textbooks."[12] They write:

> Such ineffective treatment as aspirin and/or sleeping pills, or some equivalent, prescribed with little sympathy by predominantly male physicians has now been replaced with estrogen treatment. Presumably, its apparent effectiveness in reducing the symptoms (and therefore the complaints) and ease of administration have outweighed the presence of uncomfortable and possibly dangerous side-effects.[13]

The researchers were perhaps overly harsh on the medical community when they chastised them for not evaluating the effects of estrogen—we now know that they did, albeit belatedly, for the millions of women exposed to risk. The fact does remain, however, that alternative treatments to estrogen therapy appear to have been given only cursory attention, although recently non-hormonal drugs have been demonstrated as more effective in treatment of flushing.[14]

A careful examination of the medical data on menopause also indicates that the mystique accorded the doctor—that somehow he is competent, all-knowing, and completely trustworthy—has served to shield the medical community from criticism of their assumptions about menopause. Physicians tend to rely upon their "experience," often subjective, without careful enough attention to the rigors of scientific research to enable them to distinguish between their opinion—usually based on traditional attitudes and beliefs—and the actual state of affairs. Where careful research is conducted, traditional beliefs seem to be seriously challenged.

In 1971 G. Rybo and H. Westerberg of the Department of Obstetrics and Gynecology of the University of Göteborg, Göteborg, Sweden, reported on a study that sought to investigate various biological and psychological changes that might arise during the menopause.[15] They wished to answer the questions concerning whether or not there is a specific postmenopausal syndrome—a series of symptoms to be found in women after they had reached the end of their reproductive years. Some 1,462 women, the ages of thirty-eight, forty-six, fifty, fifty-four, and sixty were examined.

During the five years following the menopause, it was found that there was a *gradual* decline in the excretion of estrogen in the urine, and a gradual change in the maturational index according to Meisel (a method of determining the level of estrogen).

But the investigators were also interested in other symptoms frequently mentioned as comprising the "menopausal syndrome." These included: palpitations, pains in the back, pains in the joints, vertigo (dizziness), headache, irritability, incontinence, weight increase, and hot flushes.

The researchers compared the symptoms of women thirty-eight years of age, who had normal menstrual cycles, with postmenopausal women forty-six to sixty years of age (the mean age of menopause in this group was 48.9 in women 54 and 60 years of age).

The results? Only the occurrence of hot flushes differed significantly between the younger women who were menstruating normally, and the women who had reached menopause. The Swedish researchers concluded: ". . . with the exception of hot flushes, there is no reason to believe in a specific postmenopausal syndrome."[16]

If the Göteborg researchers are correct, this is further evidence of how important it is for the medical complaints of women to be investigated thoroughly and not to be dismissed simply as "menopausal." Men and women at any age can have any of these complaints, and good medical practice would check them out. Indeed, many complaints of the so-called menopausal syndrome are more typical of menstruation than of menopause. The notion that there is a menopausal syndrome simply does not seem to hold up when women are viewed across cultures, in different times and parts of the world. Menopause can't be described as clearly as the symptoms of a bad cold.

As the estrogen-replacement-therapy craze grew in popularity, it embraced menopausal women in the prevailing medical tendency toward medication in general: "overdiagnosis," that is, when in doubt diagnose and treat. Still, the opposite trend, more typical of medical approach to menopause, "underdiagnosis" continued—the tendency to dismiss women's complaints as "menopausal" and emotional in nature. The dangers of both extremes are obvious. Unnecessary drugs create unnecessary problems for the body. Delay of necessary careful diagnosis and treatment of ailments are equally dangerous.

There is always the danger that a physician might carelessly dismiss the complaints of women at menopause as being but hysterical demands for attention. This danger has been recognized by the medical community as well as the women who often know that their problems are not being taken seriously. Writing, in 1973, in the prestigious *New England Journal of Medicine*, Dr. Martin J. Kelly, Jr., the Assistant Director of Psychiatry at Boston's Peter Bent Brigham Hospital, blasted doctors for dismissing women's complaints as emotional. "Sexism exists," Kelly wrote, "and it's very subtle. Physicians are also guilty of these [sexist] attitudes."[17]

K. Jean Lennane and R. John Lennane, writing in the same journal, reported on their examination of medical literature, including textbooks. They found example after example of doctors dismissing complaints as emotional, rather than treating the cause.[18]

Women at menopause are particularly vulnerable to the tendency to regard their complaints and problems as due to the vague "change of life." Mary tells of this experience. When she complained of fatigue and some dizziness, her doctor reassured her these were simply symptoms of "the change." Her weakness persisted and after she fainted at a dinner party one night, Mary sought the advice of another physician, an internist. He soon discovered that Mary was really ill, with diabetes. Fortunately, her condition improved with a changed diet.

Recently, a colleague of mine returned from work in a tropical area. Her physician dismissed her complaints as resulting from emotion at this time of life, until sophisticated laboratory tests revealed she had an amoebic infection.

A prominent woman I know, well educated and sophisticated, tells a story about an experience she had in this regard. She was thirty-four—long before she would reach menopause—and had been taking medication for a gall-bladder condition. One day she realized that she was having a bad reaction to the drug, felt that she had poisoned herself, and rushed to the nearby emergency room of a large hospital for an antidote. She was, of course, quite concerned and upset about her condition and wanted immediate care. One doctor in the emergency room said, "That might be a menopause symptom," and, turning to another doctor said, "Don't open the window, she's so nervous she might jump out."

There is no doubt, of course, that some complaints of women are not based upon organic problems, but rather upon emotional difficulties or dissatisfactions with their lives, as well as their need for attention by doctors in the absence of other ears and interested persons. The important thing, however, is that these complaints be seriously checked out for possible physical cause before flippant dismissal.

The lesson urged by the *New England Journal of Medicine* is not one for doctors alone. Women, too, share many of the notions that somehow menopause brings with it problems and these have to be endured, hopefully passing with time. The illnesses, discomforts, etc., experienced by some women at this age are, however, not innocently "menopausal." They may have nothing to do with the endocrinal changes occurring in the body—*a woman is not simply her hormones and genitalia*. Discomforts may or may not indicate other serious medical problems. The most careful diagnosis is indicated.

Women are confronted with this double-edged sword. On the one hand they live, in Western society, in a subtly sexist environment in which many physicians are influenced by attitudes that regard their complaints, especially at middle-age, as somehow influenced by the poorly defined and understood "menopause." On the other hand, the more recent years have seen a wild swing in the direction of using estrogen whether needed or not to cure or prevent a whole host of real and imagined or anticipated difficulties.

## Women Share Responsibility Too

Although physicians can be pointed to as a source of unfortunate and unnecessary medication for women at menopause, it is also true that women themselves are often the cause of this abuse.

It is well known that frequently women demand medication from their doctors, whether or not their organic conditions warrant medication. There are several possible reasons for this. An obvious one is that, given real discomfort, the requirement for alleviation of symptoms is sought and, in the absence of knowledge about possible danger, the treatment is requested. There are, however, many women who seek drugs out of a discontent with their lives; for example, women living with husbands and families that are severely restricting, in which they are monitored and controlled, or feeling somewhat useless and unimportant, who seek neurotic solutions to their discontent via medication. Such women are likely to abuse medication in ways similar to the abuse of alcohol or other drugs.

It has been suggested that such women abuse drugs for several reasons, and the use of medicine and alcohol is similar.[19] One is that the acquisition, concealment, and ingestion of medicine becomes a focus for life's activities. After all, it takes time and planning to get prescriptions, to purchase, to find places to keep or hide the medications, and to arrange for a schedule of medication. This can become the largest component of a day's work, substituting for other more realistically oriented activity.

Another explanation offered for drug abuse is that medicine, much as food for some obese persons or alcohol for the alcoholic, can be a significant source of affectional supplies. For some women, visiting the doctor, or being visited by him, receiving the attention of their family and other acquaintances can serve as an antidote to loneliness. All of us are familiar with persons whose lives revolve about visits to their doctors and concern by friends and relatives about their state of health.

Medication is also a method of some neurotic persons' assertion of their autonomy or individuality, as if by having to take medicine they assert to themselves and to others that they are special, important persons.

The taking of medication everywhere has some of these aspects attached to it. For example, the curing ceremonies of the Navajo people of the southwestern United States are characterized not only by ritual ceremonial chants and the administration of curing medicines, but also by the attentions of relatives and friends to insure the ill individual that he is important to the people around him and they wish him to be well and to continue as a participant in the society. This moral nurturance, so to speak, is an important element in his cure.

In modern society, when so many women at menopause feel either neglected, unwanted, or insignificant, it is not at all surprising to find them readily seduced by the availability and popularity of medication in this country as a solution to their ills. Far more demanding is the route of asserting their individual autonomy by dealing with their real problems, as well as the refusal to be shut out of participating actively in life around them.

Overmedication is also supported by the cultural attitudes in Western society which treat illness as a social topic of conversation, and as almost ever-present. There are many societies that do this, among them the Navajo, whose elaborate curing rituals are the subject of widespread discussion and social gatherings. Contrasted with this are those cultures, like those of the Coast Salish of British Columbia, that, though aware of illness and death, isolated their ill and rarely discussed illness as an ordinary topic of conversation, as if by avoiding discussion they would avoid trouble. On the Greek island of Delos in the Aegean Sea, in ancient times, it was even forbidden for anyone to be seriously ill and to die. The sick were made invisible by banishment to another, hospital island, and the healthy remained in their Apollonian paradise to enjoy and worship the sun.

In the Western world, one's state of health is the very first topic of conversation upon greeting—"How are you?" Perfunctory as that may be, the response often is, "Oh, I have a cold," rather than "Do you really want to know?" And, with the encouragement of drug advertisers, there is scarcely any awareness of body which is unaccompanied by some medication to anaesthetize feeling—a sneeze, a cough, a sensation in a joint or muscle, an hour without sleep at night, dryness in the throat. It is as if without medication aids to sleep, digest food, have sexual intercourse, and move our tired limbs, it would have been impossible for man to make that miraculous climb from the Rift Valley of Africa millions of years ago to the present four billion inhabitants of the earth.

Pregnancy is defined as an illness. Birth becomes a major surgical event. And menopause, experienced by all females on earth who survive into their fifties and sixties, is defined as a disease rather than a normal life process.

There is no argument with the fact that both the medicines of the primitives, many of which are unfortunately lost to our cumulative pool of knowledge, and modern medicine are extremely important and useful. Any woman who has had a bout with cystitis (bladder infection) cannot but be grateful for the rapid relief and eventual cure afforded by modern medications. Uncomfortable and unpleasant bouts with vaginitis also respond to modern drugs, with grateful thanks from women. And women whose lives have been saved by surgical obstetrics are not about to urge their sisters to forego advanced medical care. There are few indeed who would urge a return to a world without well-trained modern doctors. But the experience during the last decade, with the indiscriminate prescription of estrogens for women at menopause and beyond, points to some serious questions that have to be considered in regard to patients and their doctors and in regard to the attitudes of all toward drugs.

First of all, doctors cannot be asked to shoulder all the blame in relation to overuse of drugs in this and other countries. Both doctors and their patients are subject to the same cultural attitude that encourages medication whenever a complaint about one's state of health is voiced. There is the pervasive attitude that if something is bothering a person, there has to be a pill or potion to end the trouble —or at least the sensation of trouble.

Secondly, the barrage of propagandistic advertising by the drug manufacturers which pervades both the mass media—reaching the lay public—and the medical journals—reaching the doctors—is difficult to withstand. Sometimes doctors complain that their patients demand drugs they have heard about before the doctors—by reading the popular magazines or watching television commercials. They are faced with the problem that their patients will go off to doctors who are more "tuned in" to what is new, as if being new is necessarily better or safer. And, unfortunately, most doctors have limited time in which to engage in an educational exchange with a patient.

For women at menopause, the problems are compounded by the fact that doctors share cultural stereotypes about the difficulties of menopause, and are likely to be convinced by a patient's verbal complaint, or by their own assumptions that medication for menopause is necessary. For example, how does one measure the severity of a "hot flush"? It is unwise to assume that "hot flushes" require medication without some very careful analysis of the actual level of discomfort, yet estrogen was prescribed routinely by many to eliminate or prevent their occurrence, and the manufacturers include "hot flushes" in their ads as a reason for giving the drug.

In the same way, the patient who complains of insomnia is frequently a patient who gets her rest by sleeping till noon and who has other problems that make staying awake an unhappy experience. There is, of course, no substitute for careful diagnosis to eliminate the possibility of organic illness—the real problem arose when the assumption was made that menopause itself was a metabolic estrogen deficiency disease and that, therefore, estrogen had to be replaced as a preventive or treatment for a number of conditions that *might* arise.

Women and their doctors have also been affected by the changing practices of modern medicine. There was a time when a patient was in close relationship to the doctor, and most important, there was as a result a tremendous amount of faith in the doctor. The patient under these conditions was protected by the Hippocratic oath, taken by the doctor since ancient times, in which he pledged to help and not hurt. Many of us still share the faith that "doctor knows best."

Under conditions of modern medical care, medical practice has become highly specialized, and the relationship of the patient to the various specialists who treat the various parts of the body have become far more distant. And while a woman might trust her gynecologist, it takes more than one specialist to determine if the numb feeling in the fingertips is due to menopause or to some circulatory disturbance involving other causes and treatments. Doctors still take the Hippocratic oath, and hopefully abide by it, but the specialization and bureaucratization of medical care, while potentially able to provide vastly superior skills to the ill, also lead to the absence of close ties between the doctor and his patient as an individual whole person. Under these conditions, it is, perhaps to the benefit of the patient, more difficult to accept medication and prescriptions on faith that "the doctor knows best" simply because one doesn't always *know* the doctor. Strangers are rarely, if ever, as trusted as a person one knows cares about one.

While faith and trust play an important role in cures, either because of some psychosomatic effects or because time itself allows the body to heal, given the conditions of modern medical practice, a healthy skepticism seems very much in order. The "doubting Thomas" approach seems very wise in light of the estrogen catastrophe. Women have the right to ask their doctors for explanations concerning the drugs being prescribed, the reasons for the prescription, the alternate forms of medication available, and, perhaps most of all, a list of the drug manufacturer's statement of contraindications. All drugs, even aspirin, cannot be prescribed for all and can have negative effects or contraindications. Aspirin, for example, is not advisable for patients with a history of stomach ulcers, since it can, under certain conditions, cause stomach bleeding.

The list of contraindications for the widely prescribed estrogen drug Premarin, now indicated as a potential cause of uterine cancer when used over a period of time, ran the length of a magazine page. But this list generally appeared in infinitesimal print, on the page behind the double-spread glossy advertisements proclaiming, in bold print, the virtues of the drug.

Given the state of knowledge today, the informed, intelligent patient has the right to discuss with her doctor whether the dangers of a particular medication outweigh the dangers or discomforts of a particular complaint. She has the right to discuss the choice of treatment, including the possibility of no treatment at all.

The multimillion-dollar drug industry is not without blame in the recent wave of massive drug use. To a limited degree, in the United States there is some protection against dangerous medication. This is the result partially of the wide publicity that reports to the scientific community are given in the popular press. The level of educational reports to the readers of magazines and newspapers and to those who watch television and listen to the radio is far higher in the United States than anywhere else, and it does not take long. Indeed, sometimes it is simultaneous—as soon as some study has uncovered a danger, the local press reports it together with a scientific journal. The United States Food and Drug Administration also has advisory committees whose reports are made public and either issues warnings on use or withdraws drugs when the evidence warrants. To investigative reporters such as Ralph Nader, the FDA regulations do not appear stringent enough, and they too take on the task of keeping the public informed concerning potential or actual dangers. Congressional hearings on these matters also receive a wide press.

One such Congressional hearing by the Senate Monopoly Subcommittee in 1976 heard reports from scientists at the University of California Medical School that the protection afforded buyers in the United States did not necessarily extend to the users of the same drugs outside this country, and that the overuse and misuse of drugs abroad was of danger to Americans, as well as to the people of those countries.[20]

For one thing, the overuse of drugs abroad appears to be creating germ populations that are drug resistant, and the potential spread of these germs worldwide in this jet age could become a global problem.

Another problem which is appearing is that while the manufacturers of drugs are permitted restricted advertising in the United States—approved use according to the Food and Drug Administration regulations, and to include labeling as regards hazards—these restrictions do not apply to sales abroad where United States Federal agencies have no authority. One of the examples of the resultant abuse applies to menopausal women. This is the widespread use and sale of contraceptive drugs which are openly recommended for use in Latin America, for example, not only for contraception—an approved use—but for other conditions including problems of the menopause, for which they are not promoted in this country, and for which they present potential dangers.

While the Senate subcommittee was understandably concerned with information concerning the possible serious effects for United States citizens traveling abroad and treated by these drugs by physicians who received no significant warnings by the drug companies, the problem is obviously a serious one for the people of countries who import their medications.

As the evidence mounts, it becomes increasingly clear that faith and trust in the efficacy of drugs and the infallibility of doctors are no substitutes for intelligent, informed opinion acting as a counterbalance. It is sad to think, however, that even with the best of intentions, being well informed has become difficult for both patients and doctors now that postdoctoral pharmaceutical education is so much in the hands of the drug salesmen.

In any event, it continues to be important for all women, whether they have been on estrogen replacement therapy or not, to have regular medical checkups. It is paradoxical that woman must return to that same medical community which together with herself was sold a polluted fountain of youth—a package of pills promising "Feminine Forever" by putting her on estrogen and "Keeping Her There."

The revolt of the female body in the form of increased cancer rates is pretty good evidence that even if menopause is eventually to be found to be a metabolic disease rather than a natural process, oral estrogen replacement is certainly neither the prevention nor the cure.

There remains the very real possibility that future research may uncover the secrets of how our cells and glands are triggered to move us into the postreproductive phase of the life cycle. For the time being, efforts to interfere with this process are having effects too negative to ignore.

An approach to menopause which accepts it as part of the natural design of human life does not mean that women who do have difficulty should not be helped medically. But it does mean that for the vast majority, healthy body adjustments can be expected.

# Pregnancy and Babies

The primary biological consequence of the menopause is that women move from the ability to bear children to the loss of that ability. Still, most of us have heard, at one time or another, about "menopause babies." Can there really be such a phenomenon as a baby at menopause?

The fact is that once a woman has reached menopause it is impossible for her to become pregnant and to have a child. In the literal sense, a menopause baby is an impossibility. However, some women having skipped a menstrual period, or even several, then believe that their childbearing is over and proceed to have intercourse without contraception. Since it is possible that irregular menses are only the signs of some hormonal or ovulation changes, but not the signal that fertility is completely ended, conception and pregnancy can occur. In addition, it sometimes happens that a woman becomes pregnant, stops menstruating, and then believes that the end of her periods represent menopause. How surprised such women are when they eventually discover there's a baby inside causing their rounding figures to bulge. Sometimes these infants too are called "menopause babies."

Will these children born to women at later ages be healthy? Will the mothers be well?

## Menopause and Pregnancy

There are plenty of reasons why many women would not want to become mothers during their forties and fifties. By those years, the average woman in industrial society has raised her family and might even be a grandmother, happily welcoming a period of relative freedom from responsibility and a whole new, exciting period of her life. Husbands are likely to be older and unwilling to assume the responsibilities of fatherhood at their age.

Many people also have a sense of the impropriety of childbearing at a later age. For example, among some Gypsy groups it is considered an insult to a son for his mother to bear a child at the same time as the son's wife.[1]

But there are also many reasons why some women past forty might want to be pregnant. There are those for whom marriage has come late, whose childbearing has been postponed for one reason or another, or who simply have been unable to conceive until then. And there are those societies in which continued evidence of a woman's fertility insures against replacement by younger wives, because of the high value placed on large numbers of offspring. There are women, too, who define their own femininity and sexuality in terms of childbearing and prefer to continue to have children as long as they are able.

What are the chances for pregnancy and what are the chances for successful carrying to term?

Pregnancy is distinctly possible while the ovarian follicles continue to produce mature ovum. That possibility remains until the last menstrual period. And one can't be certain that a menstrual period is the last until at least *one year* has elapsed without a period. A few skipped months give no assurance of the impossibility of pregnancy. Nevertheless, the chances are that once premenopausal irregularity begins, not every period will represent the end of a cycle in which a fully mature ovum was produced and discharged. For that reason the chances of a conception taking place are somewhat decreased, though not eliminated, for it is the mature ovum which has to be fertilized by the male sperm before pregnancy can occur.

Once conception does occur, however, there are greater risks of a natural, spontaneous abortion occurring. This is because the changed endocrine balance in the system of the older woman affects the endometrium or lining of the womb—the reasons for the menstrual irregularities in the first place—and may interfere with the ability of the uterus to retain the fetus.

Women in their early fifties are known to have produced healthy offspring, and motherhood in the middle forties is not uncommon. Among the people of the Caucasus mountains in Soviet Georgia, women and men often marry late, and motherhood after the age of fifty is not infrequent. There is a positive cultural attitude toward such late childbearing. For one thing, femininity and sexuality are not viewed as declining with advancing age and, for another, the people of the Caucasus have a saying, "Mature parents make better children."[2]

But what are the known facts about the offspring of older women? Will an infant born to such a mother be as healthy as one born to a younger woman? While the evidence is that the vast majority of those babies will be healthy and normal, there is one condition that does appear more frequently among the children of older mothers, and that is Down's syndrome, popularly known as mongolism. The thought of bearing a mongoloid child can strike terror in the heart of any woman. A child with Down's syndrome has a variety of congenital defects which are incurable. Over a century ago, Down described these: a series of mental and physical disturbances including impaired hearing, sight, heart and circulatory difficulties, muscle, teeth, and gland problems, among others. Throughout history, the child with Down's syndrome has been an object of scorn and pity, the village idiot. The condition results from a chromosome aberration. Whereas the normal individual bears forty-six chromosomes, the Down's syndrome child bears forty-seven.

Unfortunately, the chances of a woman producing a mongoloid child increase with age. Under the age of thirty, there is one such child born out of fifteen hundred; in the early thirties, one in three hundred. But once past forty, the chances increase enormously, with one out of every forty or fifty births producing a child with Down's syndrome. As foreboding as these figures sound, that still leaves great odds in favor of having a normal child, and the people of the Caucasus are not reported to have any unusual numbers of idiots in their population. Family history plays a part—there is a far greater risk of producing a Down's syndrome infant where there is evidence that the disease has appeared in the families of the parents.

For the woman who wants very much to have a child in her middle age but has strong feelings about not having one with Down's syndrome, current medical practice has provided a way of dealing with the problem. This is the recently developed technique known as amniocentesis. Using this method, skilled technicians insert a hollow needle through the abdominal wall, into the uterus to withdraw some amniotic fluid surrounding the developing fetus. After special treatment of the fluid in the laboratory, it becomes possible to examine the cells to determine whether or not they present a normal chromosome pattern. (Amniocentesis is also used to spot metabolic problems in developing embryos, as well as difficulties children of RH negative mothers and RH positive fathers may be having.) Amniocentesis requires great skill and careful training on the part of the practitioners and should be performed only in advanced medical centers and only where it is of exceptionally great importance to the mother to know the condition of the fetus. It can induce premature labor and other hazards. For the older pregnant woman, this technique can provide her with the information needed to decide whether or not to have an abortion, if her religious scruples do not interfere.

It is not clear why Down's syndrome is more common among the children of older mothers. It may be the aging follicles or ovum. But this is just speculation—the answer is not known. The fact remains that women can have children during the early-middle years, and most of those children will be normal.

But what of the mother? What are the risks for her? If she is healthy and given good prenatal and obstetrical care, there are no extraordinary dangers of childbearing for these women. Complications arise for those women who have conditions that would increase the risk of childbearing at any age—heart, circulatory, kidney problems, etc. Since older women in general have a somewhat higher incidence of physical ailments, excellent medical care is even more essential for them. It does seem sensible, in general, for people to have their children at earlier ages. Late-middle life does not seem to be the best time, biologically, for a woman to bear children.

There is a notion that appears every now and then, and is believed by some, that to become pregnant in one's forties is an excellent way to prolong youth and postpone menopause. First, the age of menopause is not clearly related to the number of children one has had or the age of the mother when the children were born. As far as prolonging youth is concerned, the calendar does not stop with pregnancy. It is true that being pregnant is often a time of joy and beauty —two things associated with youth in this culture. Also, to be the parent of young children places one in a somewhat different social category than being the parent of grown children with babies of their own. But being pregnant can also be a physical burden for the older woman, as it sometimes is for young women, and the parent of grown children is often free to engage in the kind of activity—athletic, social, cultural—that makes her feel younger than when she was the parent of young children. Pregnancy is no magic elixir for the postponement of physical aging. Among some Moslem women of the Middle East, the ability to bear children is very important in their marriages—the end of childbearing sometimes meaning replacement by a younger wife. For such women, childbearing postpones *cultural* aging.

## Contraception and Menopause

There is nothing about menopause and the period leading up to it to physically prevent the continuation of or even the beginning of an active sex life. The chances of becoming pregnant and retaining a normal pregnancy through the delivery of an infant are somewhat decreased as a woman nears the end of the premenopausal period and menses actually end, *but* pregnancy *is* very possible indeed. A scant or delayed pattern of menstruation is no assurance to a woman that she won't become pregnant while continuing an active sex life.

Generally speaking, contraception is recommended until a year has passed after the last menstruation. "Menopause babies" are not unusual—a skipped period or two does not mean that a woman won't be fertile at various times for several years following.

Some women, who have no objection to abortion and live where legal abortions are readily available, take their chances during this period of life, resorting to this method to eliminate an unwanted pregnancy should it occur. But abortion hardly seems the wisest available method of controlling childbearing. Abortions can involve emotional complications, they interfere with the body, and they are not advisable as a regular procedure. With the many contraceptive techniques available to women, abortion seems a method of last resort.

In any event, careful diagnosis before abortion is essential for women in their menopausal years because of the irrregular pattern of their menstruation and the possibility that a delayed menstruation is not the result of pregnancy.

The most radical form of prevention of pregnancy is a hysterectomy, or removal of the womb, performed on an otherwise normal, healthy woman, just for the sake of avoiding pregnancy. There are plenty of medical reasons why this is a most unwise approach to contraception (see discussion on hysterectomy later in this book). Some doctors, hopefully reluctantly, are willing to perform this surgery for women who demand it. And there are women who "want it all out." Such women need a great deal of support and assistance by their physicians in an effort to urge them to employ less traumatic means of preventing conception.

Tubal ligation, or the tying of the fallopian tubes, is another form of surgical intervention, far less drastic than hysterectomy. In the tubal ligation operation, the passageway for the ovum to reach the womb after leaving the ovary is blocked. The male sperm is therefore unable to reach the egg, preventing conception. But, like all abdominal surgical procedures, tubal ligation does require hospitalization, and does involve some discomfort. More recent procedures, practiced in the major medical centers of the United States, have greatly simplified the operation. This operation is irreversible.

Sterilization can now be achieved by another procedure known as the laparoscopy. The laparoscope is a sleevelike instrument that is inserted into a tiny abdominal incision, spreading light over the area to be looked at. The surgeon then inserts into the laparoscope an electrical instrument with which, using heat, he is able to cauterize the fallopian tubes. The operation leaves a very small scar near the navel. Laparoscopy requires considerable skill since there is possibility of injury to the bowel or inflammation of the abdominal lining as a result. The carefully done laparoscopy, however, is an effective operation, requiring little recovery time for the patient. It is likely to enjoy a considerable vogue as women grow wary of long-term use of contraceptive pills. The long-range effects of this sterilization technique, however, are as yet unknown, and there are possible complications from the procedure.

Of course, the other surgical intervention has to do with the male. He can have a vasectomy, which prevents the sperm from being released. For a woman this would seem to be an ideal solution, for her mate to continue to be sexually active but unable to impregnate her. However, while the rate of vasectomy operations performed in the United States is rising, many men resist this solution. And many women do too. Cultural notions of potency and virility are shared by men and women. Many a willing husband has been dissuaded by his wife from having a vasectomy. While there is no relationship between the sperm and a man's ability to have erections and sexual intercourse—there are, for example, many men who are sterile for other reasons but nonetheless sexually active—there are still many people who measure a man's virility by his ability to impregnate women. Perhaps if they believed, as did the aborigines of Australia, that a man, by having intercourse with a woman, simply made room for the spirits to impregnate her, their fear of losing virility due to vasectomy would fade away. Anyway, not every man is willing to undergo vasectomy and put an end to his potential for fathering children. In many traditions, such as the Moslem, where younger wives can continue to bear wanted children, or among people with strong machismo attitudes requiring children to bear witness to male virility, women who no longer wish children must turn to methods of protection for themselves.

Aside from surgical methods of contraception, there are chemical and mechanical methods available. The chemical interferes with the body's ability to conceive or retain a pregnancy either by acting on the sperm or some aspect of the woman's body; the mechanical erects a barrier between the sperm and the ovum or between the fertilized egg and the womb.

The most extraordinary chemical method of all is, of course, the birth-control pill, which revolutionized contraception for the current generation of women. Its wide acceptance during the 1960s seemed to stimulate a whole sexual revolution—no fear of pregnancy to inhibit sexuality and more widespread extramarital and premarital sex. Of course, the pill itself cannot account for the apparent changes in mores in regard to sexuality—after all, relatively uninhibited sexuality and premarital and extramarital sex have been known to mankind throughout history and are widely accepted in cultures outside the Judeo-Christian tradition. In any event, the numbers of unwanted pregnancies were certainly reduced, family planning made more simple, and a possible aid to inhibiting the population explosion without inhibiting sex was welcomed (except for those detractors who feared a new Sodom and Gomorrah).

The pill was not an unmixed blessing for other than social reasons. Like all drugs it had its "contraindications"—reasons for negative effects on the body. It could not be tolerated by all women, especially those with heart, liver, and diabetic conditions, and evidence soon mounted that it increased chances for coronary thrombosis, embolisms, and had other side effects such as weight gain, nausea, skin eruptions, etc. For the vast majority of women taking the pill, however, its benefits in regulating conception far outweighed the minor side effects which some women had.

For middle-aged premenopausal women with irregular menses, the pill seemed fantastic. Having used other, less aesthetic forms of contraception, they now shared with their daughters the convenience of the clean, neat method of contraception that permitted "natural" sex. Some women were delighted to be "ready for any man at any time." Others were happy that "I know when I'll have my period and can plan my life. My husband and I can't take off on a holiday like a second honeymoon for me only to have my period. Intercourse is O.K. when you're menstruating, but we've always found it messy and I'd rather not. With the pill there is never such a complication." Still other women with a history of painful menstruation (dysmenorrhea) found that with the pill, for the first time in their lives, menstruation presented no difficulties.

Unfortunately, the most recent news on the pill and women over forty is not very good. Studies published in 1975 raised serious questions about the routine use of the birth-control pill as a method of contraception for women past forty. The findings were serious enough for the United States Food and Drug Administration's Obstetrics and Gynecology Advisory Committee to recommend that women over forty be urged to adopt other means of contraception.

The studies that prompted this warning report that the chances of a woman over forty on the pill getting a heart attack are greater than the chances of women not on the pill. The risk of death from heart attack appears to be more than four times as great for pill users as for non-users.

One of these studies claimed that for women in the forty to forty-four age group, the risk of a coronary thrombosis among birth-control pill users was put at 5.7 times that of non-users. Another study showed that the risk to pill users over forty was 4.7 times as great as among non-users. In actual numbers, most women who have been or are on the pill remain relatively safe—the estimated death rate for users over forty is 54.7 per 100,000 contrasted with 11.7 per 100,000 among non-users.[3] These figures do, however, serve as a warning that this method of contraception is questionable as a routine procedure for women nearing menopause. The United States Food and Drug Administration now requires that oral contraceptives be accompanied by a brochure that warns women over forty not to take the pill because of increased rate of heart attack.[4]

The reasons for this greater risk for women over forty are related to the fact that premenopausal hormonal changes are occurring in women of this age, and therefore the pill, which acts upon the hormonal balance of the body, has an effect somewhat different in these women than in those younger. It seems rather paradoxical that a woman in her early forties, often looking better, feeling more vigorous and alive than ever, often the mother of young children, and with a long life ahead to look forward to, must accept the fact that, in regard to her reproductive life, she is at the closing phase, and is therefore at greater risk, in regard to birth-control pills than are others.

And all this while she is still capable of becoming pregnant.

Fortunately, there are many alternate, safer methods of contraception available to the woman over forty. Some new, others old, none quite as simple to use as the pill. Contraceptive jellies act chemically and more safely since they do not interfere with the physiological processes of the woman's body, but do interfere with the potency of sperm. And there are the mechanical methods: the diaphragm, which should be fitted by a physician to cover the cervix, thus preventing sperm from entering the womb and usually used in conjunction with a spermicide jelly; the intrauterine loop, which is inserted by a physician into the womb, causing the rejection of the sperm. Then there are the old stand-bys—the use of a condom by the male so that no semen is injected into the vagina, and perhaps the most widely used contraceptive of all, coitus interruptus, in which the male withdraws just before ejaculation.

Of course, the safest method of all is the only truly unacceptable one—total abstinence. For those with religious scruples against contraception, the menopausal years present special difficulties. The accepted rhythm method employs a form of partial abstinence—sexual intercourse is avoided during that portion of the menstrual cycle when conception is likely to take place. Given the frequent irregularity of the premenopausal period, the rhythm method, which at best is highly imperfect, becomes most unpredictable.

The safety of the method chosen by a woman past forty insofar as the prevention of pregnancy at this time of her life is concerned is best discussed with a reputable gynecologist. The method of preference insofar as convenience, aesthetics, and enjoyment of sex, are probably best worked out by a woman and her husband or lover. It is certainly a good idea, however, to recognize that a contraceptive method used by a couple in the past may not be the most satisfactory now. For example, if a couple had used condoms or coitus interruptus, this might be a good time to experiment with other methods that might prove far more satisfactory in regard to enjoyment of sexual intercourse. There is every reason for the woman approaching menopause to search out the most desirable, safe form of contraception to insure that she and her mate enjoy the happiest of sexual relationships. And, it is generally agreed, that once a year has passed since the last menstrual period, there need be no more concern about contraception at all.

# You Don't Go Crazy at Menopause

Happily, menopause does not make women crazy. Nor need it precipitate severe emotional crises. There is no denying, however, the cultural stereotype that menopausal women are prone to depression, hysteria, etc. It's as if women cannot win—they're considered emotionally unstable and unreliable when they menstruate, and they are considered emotionally unstable and unreliable when they stop!

Among the Mangaian people of Africa, when a woman reaches menopause she is described as becoming good tempered. She is now like a man, free of all the earlier restraints imposed on her because she was a woman, now free to go and act in ways previously permitted only the men. What a different picture from that of the depressed, hysterical menopausal woman, so often depicted in our own culture.

Anthropologists know that no human condition can be described as "natural," as "inevitable," so long as there are human beings and societies that have differing customs and behaviors and values. During the 1920s, when Americans and Europeans were convinced that adolescence was necessarily a period of "*Sturm und Drang*" (storm and stress), Margaret Mead visited the Isle of Samoa, and found that there the teen-age years did not represent a stressful period of a woman's life.[1] Indeed, we know that the problems of adolescence, indeed the very definition of the period in our culture, is an outgrowth of modern industrialism. In earlier times and places children moved rather quickly into adulthood, with the accompanying responsibilities of making an economic livelihood and raising a family. Our affluent civilization has enabled more and more people for a longer and longer period of time to be "adolescent," preadult. Many of the problems we think of as "natural" to adolescence are really the result of experience in our society.[2]

So it is with the symptoms of menopause. Hysteria, depression, anxiety, if they are not universal, are best understood as one of two things. Either they are pathological conditions, due to some biological problem in those women who manifest the symptoms, or they are an outgrowth of conditions imposed by the society as women experience the transition from their procreative years to the years beyond.

One psychologist, accepting emotional upsets as "natural" to menopause, associating it with declining estrogen levels, describes the symptoms of these conditions as a

> . . . profound sense of internal inadequacy . . . reflected in the symptoms of intermittent depression or blues which appear characteristic of the menopause. The patient will complain of sudden, involuntary, easily precipitated crying spells, or a sensitivity to rejection, and an intolerance of loneliness. She speaks of a need for babying, for being cared for. She reacts with bitterness and resentment to this inadequacy she experiences within herself and often projects this self-incriminating anger and hostility onto her husband, blaming the casualness of the familiar husband for her feelings of self-deprivation.[3]

The evidence is far from clear that women who experience the symptoms described above are responding merely to a decline in estrogen levels. Indeed, about the only evidence that it is so is that giving some of these women estrogen makes them feel better. What makes one feel good and what causes the problem in the first place are hardly the same thing. The average doctor is not in a position to judge whether or not giving his patients estrogen for emotional problems is any different from other kinds of treatment—sugar-coated pills, reassurance, or a chat with a neglectful husband. It might be that the remedy proposed by Dr. E. A. Maury, the robust homeopathic French physician, in his 1975 best seller *Sognez—Vous par le Vin* (*Treat Yourself with Wine*) might have an equally uplifting effect. He recommended that menopausal women treat their complaints with four glasses of St. Emillion wine daily. Even America's own Lydia Pinkham recognized the cheering effects of her alcohol-based remedy for "female disorders."

The overwhelming majority of women, even within our own culture, do not necessarily experience emotional breakdowns during the menopausal years, despite the fact that they share declining estrogen levels with their sisters. And while the suicide rate for women is highest around the age of menopause, it remains significantly lower than that of men. While admissions to mental hospitals are generally higher for women than for men at all ages, for women the rates decline markedly in the decades past age thirty-four. And just as few would seriously propose alcoholism as a cure for the blues, so it doesn't seem wise to rush to estrogen before careful consideration of all the factors that might explain a particular woman's problems.

There is increasing research among Western psychiatrists to contradict the stereotype notion that menopause contributes to mental disorders, that emotional problems are a result of hormonal change. For example, one study of 320 psychiatric outpatients, aged eight to eighty, has found no relationship between the symptoms of the women patients and their particular age. In general, at all age levels the researchers found the women stronger than the men. In addition, there were few systematic changes in the symptoms of mental illness or the strengths that were related to age.

Writing in the *American Journal of Psychiatry*, George Winokur reports on a study of depressed women. He found that the relationship of menopause to the emotional breakdown of these women was due either to chance or to a common relationship to a third factor such as age. His conclusion was that there does *not* seem to be evidence for the traditional notion that the menopause is a causal factor in the affective disorders (depression) of women of a certain age.[4]

Explanations for the emotional problems of some women at midlife reflect differing fashions. A generation ago, in the 1940s, as more became known about interrelationships between personality and culture, explanations were sought in the effects of social relations on the life of women as they moved through the life cycle. There was a belief in "the wisdom of the body," that the body would restore its own internal balance, that the endocrine changes were normal, and that the difficulties experienced by women were imposed by a social system that cut them off from active participation and did not prepare them for an autonomous, useful life after childbearing years were over. Later, there was a resurgence of still earlier notions about the biological inevitability of the inferior position of women—although this time couched in more sophisticated terminology dealing with the physiological predestination of women's instability. Now those women who did experience problems, and even those who didn't, were to be treated with chemistry, estrogen hormone replacement, and the new tranquilizers, with a dash of psychotherapy thrown in to help women accommodate themselves to the conditions of life.

The drugs and the palliatives have soothed the troubled, but there is now a revolt against the treatment of menopause and its symptomology as if they represent inevitable pathology; a revolt by the body, in the form of adverse reactions to drugs, and a revolt by women who sense that they are well and vigorous, eager to spend this part of their life and the years ahead as active, happy, fulfilled individuals. They are unwilling and know it is unnecessary to give up their femininity, their social usefulness, or their ability to play and enjoy life. They are prepared to assume new roles, even changed personalities, as they grasp at the years stretching ahead—living fully. They are beginning to see problems in the world about them rather than in themselves.

But it is almost axiomatic in this society that when a woman past forty begins to have a case of "nerves," is jittery, and cries easily, it must be because she is in the menopause. The cultural stereotype lends itself to comedian's jokes but, more important, frequently to the neglect of the really serious emotional or physical problems a woman might be experiencing.

For example, it is entirely possible that some women reporting to their doctors may indeed be in a serious state of anxiety requiring competent psychiatric care. Yet, because they are assumed to be showing the symptoms of a menopausal syndrome, they may be dismissed with tranquilizers or estrogen, patted on the head, and told, "This too shall pass."

On the other hand, a patient complaining of the above symptoms might not be seriously disturbed at all but merely increasingly impatient with some aspect of life. The reasons for a case of the "nerves" can even be as simple as one that has actually recently appeared: apparently the ease of making coffee with the popular electric coffee makers, which churn out delicious filtered coffee in a few brief minutes, has created the opportunity for the drinking of many cups per day, inducing a caffeine "jag."

True anxiety is a mental state—as distinguished from fear—that may have a basis in reality, or sadness, which is a temporary reaction to an event or condition. The anxious patient is unable to control her condition and does require assistance. However, the average obstetrician or gynecologist is ordinarily either untrained to distinguish these conditions or does not have the time to make a proper diagnosis, or to give treatment. His primary task is, after all, to deal with the organic complaints of patients. And, in addition, he too is likely to share the cultural notion that this state is "normal" at menopause.

The etiology or causation of a patient's complaints requires careful, skillful investigation. Determining the severity of the complaints is also a difficult matter. What is a slight twinge to one person can be an intolerable pain to another. Recently, the National Institute of Mental Health has initiated a program of psychometrics, seeking to develop a method for measuring the degree of severity of anxiety and other emotional disturbances. One method of measurement, the Hamilton Anxiety Scale, developed at the University of Leeds in England, already exists. This consists of fourteen indices of anxiety to be graded by the interviewer on a scale from 0 through 1 (mild), 2 (moderate), 3 (severe), and 4 (very severe). This scale is far from precise or perfect, but it does help determine which patients require drug treatment alone or which patients may require psychotherapy, or even hospitalization. Hopefully, in the years ahead the work of the National Institute of Mental Health will devise a method whereby a patient's state can be more objectively evaluated than simply by opinion.

Emotional illness can appear at menopause, but it can appear at any time in a person's life. When it does occur at menopause it may be only indirectly related to it because it happens at the same age. There can be no assumption for any individual woman that one causes the other.

## The Double Standard

There is a double standard in regard to age, as well as to women in general, that can affect attitudes toward and treatment of the older woman with a mental breakdown or emotional problems. A very telling example of this double standard appears in the novel *Once Is Not Enough*, by Jacqueline Susann, herself a middle-aged woman when she wrote the book. In the book, the twenty-eight-year-old heroine describes her fifty-three-year-old father as "super-attractive." She also has a super-attractive lover, a fifty-seven-year-old writer, married to a twenty-one-year-old and the father of an infant son. When rejected by her lover, the heroine dashes to her psychiatrist's office. She says: "I made him give me twenty minutes, even though there was an hysterical menopausal lady waiting in the outer office. And I told him everything. And by the time I finished I was sobbing louder than the menopausal lady."[5]

The older woman's problems were automatically associated with menopause, a notion that pervades this culture. Hopefully, the psychiatrist knew better.

Fads and fashions in medicine come and go throughout history. Today's "in" drugs for emotional difficulties are the anxiolytics, drugs with a tranquilizing effect, that are composed of the compound Benzoadiazepines, which is made up of an inner ring of seven carbon atoms instead of the more common six-ring atom, and the related compound diazepam, which is known under the brand name Valium.

The tremendous popularity enjoyed by tranquilizing drugs as a treatment to allay anxiety in the second half of this century cannot be explained by pointing to the supposedly peculiar condition of menopause. The extent of this popularity is evidenced by the fact that American doctors alone wrote a massive total of 59.3 million prescriptions for one of these drugs, Valium, in the single year 1974.

Earlier, during the 1950s and early 1960s drugs marketed under the brand names Miltown and Librium became household words. Then came Valium—manufactured by the Roche Laboratories of Nutley, New Jersey, and by its Swiss parent company, Hoffman-La Roche—and the explosion into a multimillion-dollar industry. To insure popular acceptance of its new drug, Roche spent twelve million dollars for Valium advertising in 1974, or 25 per cent of the total of fifty million dollars spent by United States pharmaceutical manufacturers for all minor tranquilizers. The popularity of the drug is attested to by the fact that it captured 50 per cent of the market.

Curiously, it is reported that some Roche executives at first did not expect much of the drug but ". . . a couple of them tried it on postmenopausal mothers-in-law whom they found insufferable, and were delighted by its calming effects."[6] Assuming this is true, it tells of an incredibly crass attitude toward mothers-in-law if drugging them is seen as the way to keep them from expressing their needs and desires in life when they interfere with the convenience of sons-in-law.

In any event, despite possible unwanted side effects, Valium is a very widely prescribed drug in the world. Although women over thirty outnumber male users by two and one half to one, it is clear that women at or after menopause are not the only ones turning to tranquilizers to calm emotional states or simply to be in current medical fashion. Most of the prescriptions for these drugs are not written by psychiatrists, physicians in a better position to understand the true nature of a person's emotional state, but rather by general practitioners, who are on the whole inadequately trained in this regard, but who write 70 per cent of the prescriptions.

If so many people in the current world are "sold" on the habit of using tranquilizers, whether truly anxious or not, then millions of people share the widespread perception of emotional discomfort for which they seek relief. Women share these perceptions and fashions along with men. Yet for the woman at menopause, the cultural stereotype persists in attributing her mental state to hormonal change, while everyone else's is excusable on grounds of the vicissitudes of life.

The fact remains that should a woman at menopause exhibit the symptomology of anxiety, then she is entitled to as careful and serious a psychiatric diagnosis as is any man or woman of any age. Tranquilizers and hormones as treatment are acceptable only when medical and psychiatric diagnoses indicate.

The vast majority of women at menopause are neither anxious nor in a state of serious hormone deprivation. Yet they are forced to swim against the tide of the pressures exerted by medical fads and fashions, as well as multimillion-dollar industries that manufacture not only drugs but also a demand for them.

Many of the beliefs and observations made about personality disorders among menopausal women must be regarded with caution. Women need to recognize that many of the things that are supposed to happen to them are not necessarily so—that social pressure may define for them roles and behaviors, both in our society and others, that are neither natural nor necessary. Most women at menopause, despite any life adjustments they have to make as the years move on, remain healthy and well, their personalities unmarked by emotional breakdown—menopause alone does not cause nervous breakdowns, depression, or other debilitating mental disorders, although women of these ages do have their share of mentally ill, along with all ages and sexes in the population.

Why do these beliefs persist?

One of the explanations concerning society's negative attitude toward menopausal women has to do with the tendency for society to value order over disorder. Order, of course, has as its opposite possibility, disorder. But disorder as an ordinary and acceptable state of affairs is not generally acceptable, and only order is recognized and valued. Whoever or whatever threatens society's sense of order will thus be seen as threatening and nasty, disorderly, wrong. Women, in male-dominated societies, are seen as anomalies, threatening to the sense of order established in the male domain.[7] The expression, "You can't live with them, you can't live without them," or the attitude that women are crazy when menstruating and they're crazy when they stop menstruating at menopause are expressions of this attitude that women do not somehow fit into the order of things, that they are anomalous. They are viewed as deviants, different from the more proper male world, and manipulators who pose a danger to that world. Menopausal women in particular are thought of in these ways.

The functions of sex partners, bearers and rearers of children, while not sufficient to place women in the category of orderly things, still place younger women in a necessary category, "You can't live without them." Once her procreative powers are over, however, woman becomes more anomalous than ever. In some societies the problem is solved neatly. The postmenopausal woman is no longer a woman, she is now like a man.

The Arunta, a native people of Australia, are among those who perceive the postmenopausal women as asexual. They call older women "women father." Desexualized, the women become less threatening to men. Many of the taboos surrounding menstruation or their freedom of movement now can be lifted. No longer considered sexually available or threatening, many of the taboos preventing women from moving freely among men can now be lifted, and the older woman now has the greater freedom to come and go and speak with whomever she pleases. She is now able to do as a man and be regarded as a man. In other societies her fate is the opposite, and her social position drops very low.

Many of the attitudes toward menopause in the modern medical community are based on the limited experience of physicians with their own patients, an experience not tested against comparative analysis and careful case materials. After all, the gynecologist, as

many critics have pointed out, tends to see only a selection of cases—
those women who present themselves for treatment. If women in
their forties and fifties present themselves to gynecologists for treatment of their nervousness or insomnia, the chances are that they will
receive gynecological treatment for ailments ranging from dissatisfaction with their marriages, their children, their aged parents, their
own lives, or their neurotic or psychotic problems of earlier years.

In Western medicine, there is only a relatively recent history of association of menopause with mental disorders. One of the earliest
references was made in 1684 to the case of a woman, aged fifty, who,
six months after menopause, developed "convulsions of the stomach." In the nineteenth century physicians began to refer to menopause as frequently followed by melancholia. Diseases of the nervous
system were believed to follow in frequency diseases of the sexual organs. One writer, Heger, spoke of the nervous symptoms as: "hy-
peraesthesia, prickling and burning sensation in the skin and the
extremities, 'pseudo-narcotism,' uncertain gait, muscular weakness, insomnia, migraine, and hallucinations."[8]

By the end of the century the notion that personality disorders
were menopausal had grown to the point that Borner in 1886 was referring to personality change as the first sign of approaching menopause. Depression was one of these signs, although Borner remarked
also that in many women there was the development of a gay temperament. For others irritability and quick temper foretold menopause.[9]

It would seem that given the tremendous emphasis placed on sexuality by Sigmund Freud, as he developed his psychoanalytic theories and treatments of neurosis, he and his followers would have
paid substantial attention to the question of menstruation and
menopause. On the contrary, however, Freud all but ignores these
significant experiences of women. Menstruation is totally absent
from his 1931 essay on female sexuality, and in his work published
one year earlier, *Civilization and Its Discontents,* menstruation is
relegated to a footnote. Freud, probably in a misguided association
of the oestrus cycle of primate apes with the menstruation of females, considers that woman is at her most attractive during menstruation, but organic repression has acted to diminish the olfactory
stimuli. Freud would probably have viewed vaginal deodorants as an
extension of this into the social realm. It is this repression that he

cites as explanation for the many taboos practiced around the world against women at menstruation. The logic of this position is somewhat convoluted unless one accepts a theory of male fear of the female sexuality, since what he is saying is that because men find women so very attractive during menstruation, they erect barriers in the form of taboos or social customs, which deny the women to them!

The Freudian position on menopause is that at the end of menstruation, women re-experience the castration complex they supposedly experienced as children when as little girls they observed boys' bodies for the first time and realized girls were without a penis.

Karen Horney, who derived her psychoanalytic theories from Freud, but who, on the whole, paid far greater attention to cultural factors as they influenced the psyche, saw menstrual difficulties arising not so much from a reappearance of the castration complex of childhood, but rather from contradictory or ambivalent attitudes toward motherhood, such as fearing coitus but wanting children.

Another follower of the Freudian tradition, Helene Deutsch, has written extensively on the subject of women. Of particular concern to her has been the matter of painful menstruation or *dysmenorrhea*. Deutsch writes: "Women suffering from Dysmenorrhea assume a priori the attitude toward menstruation that all occurrences in the female genital region are an orgy of painful suffering. The physical discomfort of menstruation mobilizes and substantiates this feeling. Often a feeling of death accompanies the pain." To Deutsch this feeling is linked to a "poison" theory of menstruation which would hold that sexual activities produce poisons which menstruation then eliminates from the body. She also sees that all struggles for purification are an expression of guilt and are attempts to escape the female destiny—an essentially negative view.[10]

In a perceptive article on "The Symbolic Significance of Menstruation and the Menopause," Vieda Skulans presents some evidence suggesting that while some women do believe that menstruation cleanses the body, when viewed cross-culturally this notion is not necessarily linked to guilt, as Helene Deutsch suggests, and may, in fact, represent a positive attitude toward sexuality and foretell an uncomplicated menopause.[11]

She found that among a sample of women in South Wales, there were some who had relatively happy, satisfactory, and regular conjugal relations. These were precisely the women who complained *most* about menstruation and the need to cleanse their bodies of wastes. Skulans suggests that these women who had difficulties with menstruation were the ones who would have the most difficulties with menopause, not because of physical factors but rather because they attached so much significance to the reinforcement of their feminine roles regularly each month via purification and re-establishment of conjugal relations. The absence of this symbolic ritual required a major readjustment in their conception of their feminine roles, thereby causing menopausal problems.

On the other hand, the women who had relatively little or no difficulties with menstruation and who did not lead regular sexual lives with their husbands were the ones to have the least difficulties with menopause, since they had already undergone adjustments to their marital conditions and it was not necessary for them to do the same during menopause.

Thus, Skulans suggests that some women perceive menstruation as a regular cleansing ritual which prepares one for re-establishment of feminine sexuality in marriage, and that painful or excessive menstruation only helps to reinforce this symbolic role. The loss of menstruation at menopause throws a wrench into this rhythm, throwing the woman into a state of transition, which is difficult, until she makes a readjustment. As evidence, she cites the frequency with which South Wales women speak of how good it is to "see" them. One is reminded of the Jamaican women who refer to the menstrual flow as "health of flowers." Menopause is referred to by such women as having "lost them" or "losses."

Helene Deutsch also wrote widely on the emotional states of women at menopause and had a great influence in this regard. She refers to the time just before the onset of the menopausal period as a return of creative drives. Many women wish to be pregnant again, to have another child. She refers to apprehension concerning the "closing of the gates," as if menopause means an end to life. Yet Dr. Deutsch recognized the reality of women's problems writing, "The frequent depressions during the climacterium contain justified grief in the face of a declining world."[12] Unfortunately, little attention was paid to the fact that women everywhere in the world do not share this negative view or experience with menopause. With one third of life ahead, modern woman also is less likely to feel all is over.

Many writers have made the observation that the chief clinical feature of the depressed menopausal patient is the "menopausal syndrome." They believe that this arises from the threats to the ego appearing at this time. These threats include involution of the reproductive organs which present a token of power (castration anxiety), increased fatigue, loss of friends, economic insecurity. While unproved, even disproved, the notion that menopause causes breakdown unhappily persists.

Many women in the world become panic-stricken at the idea of their periods ending out of fear and ignorance concerning the cause. Among many people, discussion of menopause or sex in general, and even menstruation, are simply not topics of acceptable conversation. Menopause in particular is often a taboo topic. And elements of taboo are even present in our own society—women are often unwilling to admit that it is happening to themselves, often pretending and bragging about their monthly flows.

The experience of some of the women of Jamaica illustrate this. Among the rural women of Jamaica there are some who view the loss of their "health of flowers" (menstruation) with fear and lack of knowledge of the physiological causation. Often they do not seek help, despite their panic, because this subject is taboo. Most rural Jamaican women do not talk about "certain things," these things are called "private" and they are "hush, hush." To a generation of American women accustomed to television commercials of vaginal deodorants beamed into their living rooms, it may seem strange that in many places women still cannot discuss these matters openly with each other—are embarrassed or frightened about discussing them with others. For some of these Jamaican women, as it is for many rural Greek women, as well as others around the world, the fact that a woman no longer sees her menstruation can be a traumatic experience. Denial and other problems are converted into psychosomatic symptoms, often associated with hysteria. In Jamaica, for example, some women at this stage fall victim to false pregnancies. Women have been known to experience severe labor pains. Others develop neuroses or manifestations of psychotic conditions. Many have married younger men in an effort to delay aging.

The more affluent women, visiting gynecologists, receive medical help. Other women feel they are "done with the world," and turn to the church with renewed interest.

Some traditional Greek women also remain uninformed concerning physiology, and matters pertaining to sex and menopause are generally repressed and concealed. For these women the period of life between forty-five and sixty is often fraught with emotional difficulty. They are expected to be, indeed anticipate being, very irritable, troublesome, and emotionally unbalanced as well as physically ill.

Why should menopause sometimes cause difficulties and emotional problems as women make the transition of their lives from a state of childbearing ability to the many years that lie beyond? Among the Greeks, the society is very male dominated. Women are highly valued for their childbearing ability. And, in general, with cultural support going back to the horror of the Phaedra story, Greek men prefer wives much younger than themselves. Women's roles are associated almost entirely with the home, although they do, of course, work in the fields and carry on other economic activities. But their primary social roles are that of wife and mother. Traditional women were confined to the home, expected to be virgins at marriage and expected to subordinate themselves to the control of their husbands and male relatives. Their lives were subordinated to the tasks of the home.

They fear menopause, often denying it to themselves and their husbands. For many the end of menstruation means becoming old and dependent on sons and daughters. The discrepancy in age with their husbands, who are so often older, means that widowhood is not far off. Their lives, invested in children, their femininity tied in with traditional roles, seem to come to an end. It is at this time that many, like the Jamaican women, devote their energies now to the church, removing themselves from active participation in the world around them.

American women are not too different from the Greek and others who deny menopause. Injections, pills, rest cures, hydrotherapy, our responsiveness to estrogen replacements, all are sought to postpone or ward off the effects of inevitable biological change.

In part, this is due to the stress upon youth and sex appeal so prevalent in this culture. If sex and youth are synonymous with the value placed upon a person, then the threat of loss of these is distressing.

So many women have been raised, unrealistically for the modern world, to identify their personal worth almost exclusively with their looks, their beauty. Such women are, unless life develops a new resiliency, to suffer great trauma with aging.

A generation ago, the psychiatrist Lydia Sicher described the psychosomatic manifestations of menopause, which seem to aptly describe the conditions for Greek women and others who experience similar problems:

> . . . farewell to youth easily creates the frightening idea that the period between middle age and death can be scarcely anything but a time of decline not only of physical but of mental power. . . . Morbid anticipation induces states of hypochondriacal depression, a legion of physical complaints, most of which are manifestations of anxiety and anticipation.[13]

Death is often an unadmitted factor in the fears, apprehensions, and concerns of women as they reach mid-life. It is true that often they are more concerned about the health of the men in their lives, having learned that men are more vulnerable to death than are women at the same age. But concern about themselves is not absent.

All human beings, some time or other in their lives, come into confrontation with the inevitability of death—their own death. For some, deep religious faith in the hereafter, or in reincarnation helps ease the anxiety, sadness, or fear such realization provokes. For some of these, death is approached serenely, even gracefully, in the expectation of other existence. But even for these, leaving the familiar friends, relatives, and surroundings can be sad—but must be accepted and rationalized in some way.

For many others, however, the awareness of the possibility of one's own death is met with a shutting out, a blocking of continual conscious concern over the matter, as if death did not exist especially in our own case. This is easier for young people than older. Young people, although they may have had a vision of their own eventual demise, on the whole are better able to act as if death were not the inevitable counterpart of their existence. And, after all, for most it is a long way off. Some of the recklessness and even foolhardiness of the young is related to this notion of immortality. But inexorably the years, no matter how reckoned, do move us on. And eventually we reach a time when, as the sociologist Bernice Neugarten has pointed out, the years begin to be counted not so much in terms of how much time has passed since we were born, but rather in terms of how many years there are left to live.

## The Cultural View

Sociologist Ernest Becker, in a critique of Sigmund Freud and the psychoanalytic interpretation of menopause difficulties, has pointed to the social reasons for some women suffering from depression during the menopausal years. He asks the question, "Why should a woman, who to all appearances has led a satisfactory life, suddenly break down at the menopause and decide her life is not worth living?"[14] For Becker the answer lies in our social system which, he argues, has consigned women to a too narrow range of life choices or opportunities. Women whose positions and roles in life revolve completely about their femininity, including their roles as childbearers, mothers, and wives, according to this point of view, can be expected to experience difficulty. "Women become depressed in the menopause because . . . they do not have enough reasons for satisfying action, and when they lose the one apparent reason upon which they have predicated their lives—their femininity—their whole active world caves in." Defining the cause of depression in this way leads to the search for prevention of depression by creating new social roles and opportunities for women. According to Becker, "We create menopausal depression in women by not seeing to it that women in their forties are armed with more than one justification for their lives."

This sociological view of the cause of menopausal depression in some women stands in marked contrast to the Freudian approach, which searches for some repressed libidinal urge in women or in a resurgence of a castration complex. For example, Becker is highly critical of Sigmund Freud's analysis of the case of a fifty-one-year-old woman who came to see Freud because she found her life was suddenly "flooded" with an insane jealousy of a young career girl she was imagining her husband to be having an affair with. Freud interpreted the wife's problem as the result of libidinal urges she felt toward her handsome young son-in-law. Her use of jealousy language was an effort to conceal these unacceptable feelings from her conscious level of thinking.

Becker, in reanalyzing the case, argues that it makes more sense to recognize that this fifty-one-year-old woman had invested her life in the wife and mother role, and now finding herself with declining beauty and no children, she sensed her declining value to men, particularly her husband. Unable to express her feelings of rage at this new state of lessened importance, "without words in which to frame her protest," the protest against helplessness and potential meaninglessness took the form of jealousy accusations.

It is difficult, today, for us to know all the possible ramifications of this particular woman's experience and problems. It could very well be that her husband *was* having an affair with a young career girl, that her feelings of jealousy were based upon a real situation—one she could not bring herself to face openly—and the possibility that she was losing her husband's love and concern to another, more desirable and interesting woman. To become somewhat depressed or angry or jealous in this situation is not unreasonable.

The fact remains that how a woman reacts is not necessarily out of some amorphous mysterious entity called "menopause." She reacts out of her past experience, out of her personality strength, which has developed over a lifetime, and out of the variety of choices open to her which keep her from feeling trapped, imprisoned, as it were, in only one position upon which her entire well-being is dependent. That any woman who has invested her life in a relationship with a husband should feel threatened at the possibility of his leaving, whether real or imagined, should hardly be surprising. But to enter into a state of depression is an expression of helplessness and hopelessness on the part of those women who feel no value in and of themselves outside of a narrowly defined feminine role; dependent on their beauty and ability to bear and raise children, unprepared to deal with the modern world as autonomous, independent individuals. And for many women the world out there is cold and uncaring, making even the competent woman feel unwanted as she ages. It takes a lot of courage and strength to withstand the withering effects of a rejecting world.

The prevailing questions remain whether or not the emotional problems and psychosomatic ailments faced by some women at this period of their lives are a direct result of hormonal changes within the body, or whether they are the result of changing social conditions affecting the older woman, as well as possibly the manifestations at this age, in heightened form, of previously existing psychoneurotic conditions. Thus, again we are confronted with the nature-nurture controversy: Is biology woman's destiny, inevitably causing some women to be "crazy," or is culture so arranged to confront women with both the self-fulfilling prophecy that they will experience emotional breakdown and create those conditions that cause it?

The evidence pointing to biology is far from conclusive. While estrogen made some disturbed women feel better, so do other drugs used on persons at all age levels. And the scientific studies required to improve our understanding of the physiology of aging remain yet to be done. The association of breakdown with age is no evidence that the physiology of menopause itself is at fault—although with so much as yet not understood the question must remain an open one.

Still, the laboratory of human experience throughout the world seems to point in other directions, to the conditions of life experienced by women in different social settings throughout the world. For menopause is not simply a biological change of life. In many places and times it represents a social change of life as well. And again, the experience of mankind is that a social change of life need not be one of despair and gloom. The period of life during and after menopause can and does represent for many women around the world the high points of their lives—with all aspects of their lives enhanced, the inhibitions imposed by their cultures released to permit them improved participation in sex, high social status, and social participation.

# Middle Age and Health—Women Are Mortal

The best news about menopause is that we are now in a time when, more than ever before in the history of the world, women are living to experience it. The average length of life is increasing, not only in the advanced countries of the world practicing sophisticated medical technologies, but as a worldwide phenomenon. Death rates are falling off sharply, and the later one was born the longer the life expectancy.

The experience of the City of London is dramatic in this regard. In 1849 there were 69,000 deaths in London. In 1973 deaths were up to 89,000, but the population of London had jumped from 2,400,000 to 7,300,000! The death rate had declined over 44 per cent in little more than a century. These remarkable gains are continuing into this generation of middle-aged persons. For example, in the United States, the death rate for persons forty-five to fifty-four was 12.2 per 1,000 in 1920, and dropped a striking 42 per cent to 7.2 by 1970. People fifty-five to sixty-four experienced a death rate of 23.6 per 1,000 in 1920, and that number dropped 30 per cent to 16.6 in 1970.

And women continue to outdistance men in the push for survival. In the United States the average life expectancy for women in the mid-1970s was eight years greater than that of men—75.9 years compared with 68.2. Women have, in this country, experienced the most notable gains in survival.[1]

Of course some women have always survived into middle and even very old age. The increased percentages today are largely due to the fact that fewer children and young people now die of the infectious diseases that plagued populations in earlier times to a far greater extent than they do in the modern world. Infections and plagues have not left us, and every now and then the outbreak of a lethal disease reaches the headlines of newspapers and provides gruesome reminders that infection is still with us. But these were hardly news in the past; they were everyday occurrences. Thanks to improved nutrition, public sanitation, clean water supplies, and sewage disposal systems, our survival rates have jumped. Antibiotics and inoculations have played their role as well, although increasingly the credit for improved longevity is given to those improvements in conditions of life that have helped wipe out the occurrence and spread of disease to begin with. For example, antibiotics may fight childbed fever, enabling a woman to survive childbirth, but sanitary hospital conditions and sterilized procedures prevent infection from occurring in the first place.

The projections for continued long life are also dramatic. Currently, in the United States, almost 30 per cent of the population is between forty and seventy years of age. Those over seventy constitute 6.5 per cent of the population. By the year 2030, if current birth trends continue, it is estimated that 17 per cent of the nation will be over sixty-five years of age![2]

The biological and social consequences of the increased longevity as well as population shifts to a larger proportion of older people are far reaching.

Never before in the history of the world have so many women been able to look forward to one third of their lives to be lived beyond the period of their reproductive functioning. To live out those added years in good health and well-being as a constructive member of society is the challenge of our time. If once it was said life begins at forty, today it can be said that fifty and even sixty are years that hold the promise of continuing growth, experience, and joy. But they can also be years of wear and tear—fraught with physical breakdown of the body, and filled with the despair of loneliness, the impact of changing values all about, and the dangers of too early retirement, without choice, from sexuality and from social and economic participation.

We pay a price for prolonged life but, as the saying goes, better that than the alternative.

Women have some health problems specifically related to their sex, but in general, they share with men the complaints common to all persons of the same age level who have survived their youth and early adulthood. And, while survival rates continue to rise, the facts of life are that chronic ailments may, for some, cause a degree of limitation of activity the older one gets. Most people remain well and able to continue full activity. Even among persons over sixty-five, only 15 per cent of those chronically ill report themselves so severely handicapped that they are unable to carry on major activity whether outside the home or housework. And even these figures may be somewhat inflated as insurance and welfare plans carry a bonus for permanent disability. Unfortunately, if disability is worth money, some are likely to claim it, justifiably or not.

Women between the ages of forty-five and sixty-four share with men those common complaints that come with age: arthritis and rheumatism (it does get harder to do somersaults); heart trouble, more prevalent among men, however; and back and spine troubles. "My aching back" is no longer a joke when it gets harder to get up after sitting in a chair any length of time. Men and blacks are much more prone to hypertension and high blood pressure, than white women at these ages.

The incidence and prevalence of certain diseases accelerate during the middle years, but this is especially so after the age of fifty-five— the menopausal decade of forty-five to fifty-five showing some increase but not an especially marked one.

Women, generally, are less ill than men,[3] the only major illness in which rates are higher for women is diabetes. The male rate for heart disease is consistently two or three times the female rate—women have to face up to the reality of a future possibly devoid of a husband or lover. Hypertension is also on the increase, again for men more than women. This may be a reflection of the survival of more young people into the older age brackets—it may also be the result of the tensions and strains faced in modern society, particularly by men and possibly related to the requirement that they be successful, aggressive, and achieving.

Problems with eyes, hearing, etc., also increase, again with men bearing the brunt of the increased rates of disability.

Women after forty, including the menopause decade of forty-five to fifty-five and beyond, may be more beautiful, feel more sexy, more strong and assured than ever before. They may respond eagerly to the adage "You're not getting older, you're getting better." That is a fantastic, positive attitude to have, but it is only partially related to reality. Life can be glorious, and one can feel as healthy and vigorous as ever before. The facts, however, are that the older one gets, the greater the chance of developing some illness or disabling condition. And what it also means is that attention to one's health and good medical care, aside from all the other social ramifications of an aging population, become more important than ever.

And that terrorizing enemy, cancer, continues to lurk—where and when it might strike, a big question mark for all. For women aged forty-five to fifty-four, cancer of the breast and cancer of the womb rates go up. Men, and now more women, become prone to cancer of the lungs and bronchus. After fifty-five the rates of breast cancer continue to increase; men have their continuing high rates of lung and bronchial cancer, and now prostate cancer rates among men also go up.

Essentially what is happening is that, on the whole, the infectious diseases have been pretty much conquered—the World Health Organization doesn't even recommend smallpox inoculations any longer. And now, as more and more people survive into middle and older age, medicine must turn its attention to the problems, many of them chronic, which seem to arise as we move into the later phases of life.

For women this may or may not be a bonus. Menopause, especially, has been a neglected phase of medical research and attention. And too often women have been dismissed as simply nervous menopausal ladies when complaining of real physical problems. But this is no longer a realistic approach. With more women living longer and longer, they are a necessary concern for medicine, and hopefully many of the conditions we now think of as normal with aging will be found to be as unnecessary as the measles. But at the same time as medical concern replaces the frequent *laissez faire* attitude of under-treatment that prevailed in the past while greater attention was bestowed on the gynecological problems of younger women, new attentions may sometimes lead into strange pathways and cause unnecessary damage. The estrogen fiasco of the 1960s and 1970s in which women, many of them upper-middle class getting the "best" medical care, were fed estrogen to forestall the impediments of aging is an example—it was later found that estrogen led to the danger of increased uterine cancer. Remedies and approaches to the aging process are neither simple nor readily available. Women must be protected from undue harm caused by overly eager purveyors of drugs and dreams.

Women at menopause are justifiably concerned about the real threats to their health posed by disease. Life grows increasingly precious and fragile the older one gets. To be able to fill the second half of her life with experience, with growth and fulfillment, she knows requires her health. And health is increasingly difficult to take for granted.

A woman is especially concerned with certain ailments at menopause—will she now have heart trouble, new gynecological problems, breast cancer, and a myriad of other unwanted biological disasters? How can she avoid them? How can women retain the vigor to live a full and happy life which is becoming increasingly possible as life expectancy keeps growing longer?

## Heart Attacks

It is popularly believed that while they are still menstruating women are protected from coronary heart disease as compared with men. This protection is usually attributed to the fact that the estrogen in women's bodies lowers the cholesterol content of the blood.

Does this mean then that with menopause and its accompanying lower level of estrogen production, women's susceptibility to heart disease increases? Does this imply that estrogen replacement is advisable in order to protect against this eventuality? The evidence is heartening—all women are not about to have heart attacks because of the lowered production of estrogen coming with the onset of menopause. And there is no evidence clearly indicating that estrogen replacement, a potentially dangerous procedure, protects against heart attacks. What are the facts?

First of all, unfortunately, there is an acceleration in the rate of coronary artery disease for both men and women that is correlated with increase in age. This rate of acceleration *does not change* during the menopause. The older you are, the greater your chances, and menopause is only one segment of that life cycle. It is known that men do have more heart attacks than women. Studies in Finland showed a rate of 10:1, studies in the Netherlands showed a rate of 9:1, *but* these rates declined in the fourth decade of life, in advance of the menopause. The change in ratio was due not to the fact that the rate for women went up but rather that the rate for men declined.[4] The decrease in the male-female ratio of coronary artery disease mortality that comes in the fifth decade of life is principally due to a lower rate of acceleration of male mortality—the men have had their dangerous years already—rather than to any menopause-induced increase in the rate of acceleration of female coronary disease mortality.

It is also known that the sex difference in coronary heart mortality is much smaller or negligible in populations lacking the "affluence" and "high standards of living" of the United States and other Western nations. For example, in the forty-five- to fifty-four-year age group, in 1950, the ratio of male-female coronary death rates was 5 to 1 in the United States, 2 to 1 in Italy, and slightly greater than 1 to 1 in Japan. The difference in coronary heart disease mortality between men and women is very much less among blacks in the United States. Among black women in the United States, the average age for first myocardial infarction (heart attack) was fifty-six years. Among white women the mean age at first myocardial infarction was 66.5 years.

The lower coronary artery disease death rates in women are, in the United States at least, limited to the white population; seen in affluent societies, especially in the United States and Europe. Lowered rates do not apply to women who have complicating disorders such as diabetes and hypertension. A prior medical history of poor health, especially diabetes and hypertension, is conducive to a greater chance of having coronary difficulty all through life. The fact that women in their premenopausal condition produced estrogen does not protect them from the coronary artery disease that can lead to heart attacks, where there are predisposing disease factors.

Estrogen has been given credit for many things. It is supposed to protect the female from the dangers of high-cholesterol blood levels, which themselves are indicted as a cause of coronary heart disease. If estrogen production declines during the menopause and ends with it, one way to counteract high cholesterol and the dangers associated with it would seem to be to administer estrogen. *But* scientific studies show that the administration of estrogen to men and post-menopausal women *does not alter the body's ability to handle cholesterol*. The lipidlipoprotein pattern, which does this, does not return to the premenopausal state with the administration of estrogen. Besides, an increased vulnerability to coronary difficulty and blood-clotting irregularities are associated with estrogen administration.

Some surveys of medical and autopsy records have been made, but these do not establish a protective effect of estrogen or ovarian function against coronary artery disease. Several studies appear to document that postmenopausal women, or women with artificially induced menopause (surgical removal of organs), do show evidence of greater coronary difficulty. *But* these studies are generally based on records that were not kept with a consistent standard of reporting, and their authors are wary about concluding that absence of estrogen was the predisposing factor in the disease. Also, the studies group those with artificial menopause, generally induced because of some disease factor to begin with, with those women who have had a normal spontaneous menopause. It is the normal with which we are primarily concerned here.

It would appear, on the basis of the most recent scientific evidence, that the lowered vulnerability to death from coronary heart disease enjoyed by affluent white women is either unrelated to ovarian function or is related to some aspect of the ovarian function not yet discerned. The shifts in the balance of sex hormones that have been suggested as influencing heart attacks among men is opening new avenues of research for understanding the very complicated processes of the human body. Until more is learned about body chemistry the best guarantee against heart difficulty seems to be protection against infection, appropriate nutrition, no smoking, heredity, avoidance of unnecessary drugs, and exposure to whatever non-polluted air is available.

## Menopause and Breast Cancer

When within a period of a few weeks both the wife of the President of the United States and the wife of the Vice-President underwent mastectomies (removal of the breast), the women of the United States descended en masse to physicians' offices for examinations, as they were dramatically made aware of the frightening prospects of breast cancer.

Both Betty Ford and Happy Rockefeller are women in their middle years, and while all women suddenly developed a consciousness of their state of health, middle-aged women were understandably wondering about whether or not they experience any peculiar susceptibility to the disease.

Unfortunately, in the case of breast cancer as with all cancers, there is as yet incomplete understanding and agreement on the cause, prevention, and treatment of this dreaded disease. It is known, however, that the rate of breast cancer does increase steadily with age—the older one is, the greater are the statistical chances of occurrence. Some investigators point to the interesting phenomenon that there appears to be an interruption in this rate of increase precisely around the age of menopause! For premenopausal women the risk of breast cancer increases steeply with age. Among women of the same age, those who are postmenopausal women have a lower risk of developing breast cancer than those who are premenopausal. Speculation on the cause includes the hypothesis that there may be more than one cause of breast cancer, such as one relating to the physiology of premenopausal women, which declines with the rate of estrogen production, and one related to the physiology of postmenopausal women, which is related to the development of androgen (a male hormone) dependent tumors.[5]

Examination of the data on breast cancer also points to the fact that women who have experienced premature, artificial menopause due to surgery at a relatively early age seem to have a lower risk of breast cancer.

These facts have led to the suggestion that "Hormone therapy to delay the menopause would be predicted . . . to give an increased risk of breast cancer during the time that menopause was delayed."[6] In other words, the menopausal woman is at no special risk during this period of her life other than the risk ordinarily associated with aging: that interference with hormones was likely to increase the risk.

Once again the advocates of hormone replacement therapy are back in the picture. It was widely claimed during the early 1970s that estrogen replacement gave an added measure of protection *against* breast cancer. But in 1976 Dr. Robert N. Hoover, head of the environmental studies section of the National Cancer Institute, called the studies showing that the substances protected women against breast cancer as "meaningless," and indicated that the National Cancer Institute had data to show a link between estrogen compounds and breast cancer.[7] Evidence is mounting that the predicted dangerous effects of estrogen in relation to breast cancer among some postmenopausal women are being confirmed. Now the considered opinion of the medical community is that routine prescription of estrogen during or after the menopause is inadvisable, as opposed to short-term treatment for vasomotor complaints such as severe hot flushes or for atrophic vaginitis. The U. S. Food and Drug Administration now requires that birth-control pills—all of which contain estrogen—be labeled as inadvisable for women past the age of forty.[8]

Most women do not get breast cancer, whether on medication or not. But all women must take into account the possibility of its occurrence. The misfortune that befell the two leading ladies of America was, because of the vast publicity that accompanied their experience, a major lesson for all. Every woman requires regular physical examinations including that of her breasts. Most examinations include palpation, but the newer method of mammography, in which a picture of the breast tissues is taken, provides the possibility of earlier diagnosis. However, routine mammography for all women has been questioned recently as unnecessarily exposing healthy women to the damaging effects of radiation. The method is, nevertheless, useful in diagnosis when suspicion of a growth exists.

It is also wise for every woman to learn from her physician, or from a clinic set up to teach, the techniques of self-examination, permitting the possibility of more frequent checkups. The checkups must continue regularly through a woman's life. Menopause gives neither any special danger, nor does having passed menopause protect one from breast cancer; the rates continue to go up with age. Betty Ford's condition was uncovered during a medical examination; Happy Rockefeller reported that she discovered her condition upon self-examination. The one-shot rush to their doctors by millions of American women as a result of the illness of these two public figures confirmed for most that they were healthy. But, again, this confirmation must continue to take place on a regular basis throughout life.

Early diagnosis and treatment has greatly increased the survival chances of women with breast cancer. The method of treatment is best decided upon by a woman and her physician. There is controversy about treatment, and women have a right to be informed about the extent of their condition and alternate forms of treatment if they wish. Breast cancers vary in type and extent of spread. Surgery can vary from simple excision of the tumor; to removal of the breast; through, in a more radical mastectomy, removal of the breast, portions of the pelvic wall, and the surrounding glands. Treatment may involve irradiation, and chemotherapy to destroy cancer cells in the blood stream and lymphatic system.

What about the emotional trauma of mastectomy? There are, of course, some women who have emotional reactions to operations like hysterectomies in which the very core of a woman's feminine organs are removed. But the womb is hidden deep within—and not visible to the eye. The breasts are everywhere in this culture presented as the symbol of femininity, staring at one not only from the centerfold of *Playboy*, but displayed in alluring postures on the pages of the daily newspapers and family magazines. And how will a husband or lover react? A woman is, understandably, perhaps firstly concerned about her state of health, but, beyond that, her appearance and presentation of self as a woman and lover are justifiable concerns in a culture that places such an emphasis on the bosom as sexual allure.

Fortunately, the matter of public appearance presents no problem. The very manufacturers of the undergarments and clothes designed to heighten beauty for all women have worked their magic so that the woman with mastectomy appears as whole as ever—indeed, she is hardly the only one for whom garments enhance or even give illusions of smallness, depending on the current fashion. Although the procedures are still controversial, new efforts are being made by plastic surgeons to reconstruct breasts after mastectomy, using silicone implants.

What about her husband? What if she is single and wishes to marry, or remarry? Will men be attracted to her? First of all, mastectomy does not mean a woman does not wish to continue or even begin an active sex life. Indeed, the shock of this brush with destiny can cause in some women an intense desire to enjoy life. Where a good love relationship exists, it is founded upon more than the physical presence of the breast. If problems arise in a marriage, some counseling is advisable. Researchers at the Long Island Jewish Hillside Medical Center have found that in most situations in which women have difficulties with their love life, there is no real difficulty in the actual experience of making love. Sometimes, however, there is a barrier in the mind—of the woman—that she is no longer desirable. It is unnecessary, however, for desirability to be a function of the breast. There is a whole body and a whole person. Feeling at ease with one's self is an important adjunct to desirability. Still, some women who have had mastectomies find that while they are ready to go on as before, occasional social prejudice against them exists in society—some employers even denying them jobs. Women are increasingly refusing to be treated in this manner.

The American Cancer Society maintains a Reach to Recovery program which puts mastectomy patients in touch with other women who have had this surgery. Sharing experience, insights, and positive approaches can help the new patient through a period of adjustment.

## Atrophic Vaginitis

One condition of the vagina associated with the postmenopausal state is known as atrophic vaginitis. It does *not* occur among all women, and it can occur at any age. The symptoms of this condition are not unlike that of other forms of vaginitis; they include discharge, itching, burning, and dyspareunia (painful intercourse). The vaginal discharge often is blood-tinged, and the vagina itself shows small areas of superficial hemorrhages. While this condition can be accompanied by vaginal infection as well, atrophic vaginitis is really the result of the disappearance of the glycogen-containing superficial cells of the vaginal epithelium (lining) which occurs with the withdrawal of estrogen.

Being at menopause does not mean that a woman necessarily is about to get this type of vaginitis. For one thing, it has been shown that some estrogenic function remains in the majority of women for at least ten years past menopause. Severe atrophy is found in only 20 to 25 per cent of women within a ten-year postmenopausal period, and in only 37 per cent of patients after ten years.

For those women who *do* develop vaginal difficulties directly related to estrogen deficiency, there is rapid help available. An estrogen-containing cream applied to the vagina over a two-week period, and voilá—the vagina is returned to its former condition, with the glycogen content of the epithelial cells restored as well as normal flora. A weekly application maintains the vagina in its youthful condition. There are alternate forms of treatment as well that can be discussed with the gynecologist. Since this is a local treatment, it does not seem to hold the danger that oral estrogen does. For the majority of women who do eventually develop this condition then, atrophic vaginitis occurs past menopause and is readily corrected.

## Urinary and Vaginal Complaints

Urinary and vaginal infections are not unusual during the menopausal years. However, it must be kept in mind that these complaints can occur in women at any time in their lives, and their occurrence during menopause requires as careful treatment and concern as would be given to younger women. They are not necessary conditions, and no woman at menopause should expect that these problems will simply pass with the years or that they are simply things she must learn to live with because there is little one can do about them.

Infections are conditions that can occur irrespective of age or sexual activity. Little girls commonly have pyelitis—an infection of the urinary tract—years before they menstruate or engage in sexual relations. The very anatomy of the female body lends itself to infection in these areas. The proximity of the urethra, vagina, and anus and the secretions in the area create a tendency toward moisture and warmth, creating excellent conditions for the breeding of bacteria. The recent tendency toward wearing nylon underpants, nylon pantyhose, tight-fitting trousers frequently made of synthetic materials that are not porous, has been indicted by many in the medical profession for increasing the amount of infections precisely because heat and moisture are retained. Other causes of infection include exposure from an infected sex partner; injury to tissues from accident or especially active sex; change in tissues due to estrogen deficiency; lowered resistance in the body due to some other ailment; and the possible change in body chemistry or destruction of beneficial bacteria due to the taking of medication such as antibiotics for an ailment elsewhere in the body.

The most common of the urinary infections are urethritis (inflammation of the urethra, the urinary tube leading from the bladder) and cystitis, which involves infection in the bladder. Any woman who has experienced these common ailments knows how uncomfortable and frightening they can be, even though both respond readily to modern medical treatment. Symptoms of both include painful, frequent urination, with a burning sensation. The symptoms of cystitis are more dramatic in that they also include, often, intense urgency, spasm upon urinating, as well as blood in the urine.

Both of these conditions respond almost immediately to the administration of preparations designed especially for urinary tract infections.

It is extremely important that any urinary infection be completely eliminated. The very best medical care would include not only careful examination to eliminate other possible causes of the symptoms, it would also include a culture of the urine to locate the specific organism responsible for the infection. Although the dramatic symptoms of the illness are removed quickly with medication, they are likely to reappear—chronic cystitis is not unusual—unless the infection is completely removed, which may include up to four weeks of medication, as indicated by a urine culture that is infection free and the conditions that predisposed the woman to the illness are corrected.

Before modern medication women with these illnesses were treated with baths and bed rest. Warm baths still serve to make the infected woman feel more comfortable, as well as help release retained infected urine. Even today, the Greek Government tourist brochures advertise certain islands with their hot springs as being particularly valuable for women with gynecological and urinary ailments.

While on medication a woman is advised not to drink any alcohol and to go easy on the tea and coffee. Sexual intercourse is best delayed until healing has taken place—ordinarily it would be too painful given these conditions anyway.

Even a woman who has never had urethritis or cystitis while young is likely to experience the infections by the time she reaches middle age. Sometimes exceptionally active sex, or sex after a prolonged period of abstinence, can irritate tissues and predispose them to infection. The term "honeymoon cystitis" is used to euphemistically describe this. "Honeymoon cystitis" can occur at any age. But the menopausal woman is also likely to be experiencing changes in her tissues which also predispose her to infection.

There are, fortunately, several things which can be done to prevent urinary tract infections. Elimination of sex is happily not one of them. There is no reason why sex life should not continue. Careful hygienic methods are essential, however. Regular bathing, regular douching according to a gynecologist's recommendation (disagreement concerning the necessity of douching continues)—vaginal infections can spread into the urinary tract—and, perhaps most neglected of all, drinking a great deal of water. So many women have the misguided notion that if they drink a great deal of water they will become bloated, not lose weight if they wish to, and generally just not look trim. The retention of water by body tissues is not the result of how much water one drinks. People with kidney disease or heart disease have difficulty in removing water from the body, but the normal individual will either excrete the water through the bladder and urethra or through the skin via perspiration. Two quarts of water a day in the normal person will help inhibit infection. This is especially necessary in warm weather and dry climates. Some doctors also recommend that whenever on any antibiotics, patients eat yoghurt to replace beneficial bacteria being destroyed along with the illness-producing ones in the body by the medication. (*Pasteurized* yoghurt doesn't help.)

## Osteoporosis

Osteoporosis is one of those unhappy conditions that is often cited as one of the dread consequences of menopause, although most women never get it to a serious degree. Basically, since it is a condition of decalcification of the bones, it is the disease that brings to mind the picture of the old woman, shriveled in stature, with severe joint pain, and subject to multiple fractures.

It is estimated that some four million persons in the United States have a significant degree of osteoporosis,[9] the estimate escalating to as high as twelve million in the ads of the estrogen manufacturers, who have urged the prevention of osteoporosis among women by the routine administration of estrogens.

The disease is diagnosed by X-ray evidence of bone decalcification; as well as by decrease in stature; kyphosis (curvature of the spine); and severe joint pain, which appears late in the course of the disease. In very advanced conditions, the fragile bones give way, break, and lead to serious falls. Often the broken hips of elderly persons are caused by this condition rather than by the falls which result. But these symptoms appear usually among the very aged, rather than younger women, and evidence of significant osteoporosis more frequently does not appear until ten years after the cessation of the ovarian function.

Since no one looks forward to experiencing the ravages of clinical osteoporosis, or even mild forms of the disease, the question of whether it is possible to prevent it from occurring, or how to treat it when it does occur assumes great significance.

Again, unfortunately, we are once more dealing with a condition that is easier described than understood. The precise metabolic defect that leads to the disease is imperfectly known, and treatment, therefore, varies according to the particular theory or explanation believed.

Going along with the popular notion that the decrease in estrogen can be blamed for most menopausal ills, the last decade saw the popularity of routinely prescribing estrogens in menopausal patients for prevention or treatment of osteoporosis. And it did appear that estrogen was working its miracles as evidence grew that estrogen helped to maintain a normal calcium and phosphorus balance, preventing loss of calcium from bones. Also, experimental studies confirmed the clinical observation of physicians that their patients with demonstrated osteoporosis improved dramatically, with their painful symptoms relieved under a regimen of the hormones stilbestrol and progesterone, or ethisterone.

But treating patients with advanced states of a painful illness and routinely giving a drug as a *preventative* for a disease that might not appear are two different things. And hormone therapy has come under serious question as regards osteoporosis, as it has for other things as well. Aside from any unwished-for side effects or dangers of the drugs, it is clear that although symptoms were alleviated, X-ray evidence of changes did not show up, although some investigators suggest the results may take upwards of ten years before demonstrated by X ray.

Also, other theories of osteoporosis, as well as the known dangers of routine hormonal administration, suggest that it is not advisable for the healthy woman to use estrogens to prevent osteoporosis.

One of these theories argues that bone density in both men and women decreases with age and at a steady rate not, apparently, related to any one event in the life of a woman, such as menopause. Also, it has been noted that prolonged immobilization for any cause, such as confinement to bed for several weeks or months, is followed by osteoporosis, despite diet or hormonal administration. These suggest, then, that use or exercise represents the best way to increase the density of the bones. One major gynecology text suggests, "Perhaps a game of tennis or jogging once around the block, if other more productive facilities are not at hand, is a more effective way of maintaining bone density in aging women than steroid therapy."[10] Aside from exercise in her later years, women are also well advised to continue a nourishing diet.

Medical disagreement about significant osteoporosis continues, with some claiming it to be an uncommon disease with a complex cause involving nutritional, physical, and metabolic factors, and others arguing that it is widespread and requires routine preventative treatment.

But, even before the recent exposure of the dangers of hormonal replacement therapy for all women, the *Medical Letter on Drugs and Therapeutics* announced that

> . . . in the opinion of a majority of *Medical Letter* consultants there is no convincing evidence that estrogen administration reduces the loss of bone mass in aging women. Symptoms attributable to osteoporosis may be estrogen-responsive, but placebo effect could be important in such relief. Calcium balance often becomes positive early in the course of estrogen administration in osteoporotic patients, but long-term treatment is accompanied by a less positive, or return to a negative, calcium balance.[11]

Routine administration of estrogen to healthy women was not recommended.

Any medical textbook can recite a litany of ailments that might befall women as they age. Men have their health problems also. The fact of the matter is that most people stay rather well, their physical complaints are modest, and only in the case of a minority of people cause any significant interference with their ability to pursue an active life. Without a doubt, a full life in the middle years and beyond is easier to achieve given the foundation of a healthy body. With a little bit of luck, women have lots going for them in this regard.

# Hysterectomy—The Chances Are
# You Won't Need One

Twenty-five to 30 per cent of American women aged fifty to sixty-four have had a surgical menopause, most commonly as a result of hysterectomy. Why do so many women have hysterectomies? Why especially at menopause?

It would be nice to be able to answer this question by the simple and obvious answer, "Because they need them"—need them to save their lives or to prolong their lives or to make their lives significantly more comfortable. To some extent these reasons do account for many hysterectomies, but not by a long shot all of them. There is curious variation in the rate of hysterectomy from place to place. In the United States a woman living in the South or the West has a greater chance of having the operation than a woman living in the Northeast or North Central states—the rate is almost 50 per cent higher in the South than in the Northeast. Rates vary from state to state and within different sections of the states.[1] In Canada, between 1967 and 1971, the rate in British Columbia was 13 per cent above the national average; in Alberta, 30 per cent above; while in Manitoba it was 25 per cent below, and in Ontario, 20 per cent below.[2]

Now the gynecological problems of women can't be that different from place to place. Problems of the womb are not as clearly associated with environment as is something like lung cancer rates which are associated with working environment, air pollution, and cigarette smoking. What is turning out to be the obvious and increasingly documented cause is the variety of medical practice. And it is not simply that more operations are being performed because they are needed, but that more operations are being performed and a large number of them are not needed. The situation has reached such proportions that the medical profession itself has become very concerned and begun to institute methods for reducing the amount of unnecessary surgery. The American College of Obstetricians and Gynecologists is formulating stricter standards and criteria for performance of hysterectomy, and the Joint Commission for the Accreditation of Hospitals, the health profession's voluntary accrediting body, as well as governmental agencies now require stringent evaluation procedures concerning medical practice in order for a hospital to maintain accreditation. Labor unions and medical insurance companies are beginning to encourage, even require, second opinions before their members undergo elective surgery.

Hysterectomy is a radical procedure, and it is *irreversible*. Once the organs have been removed there is no way of replacing them. For women of childbearing age this would seem to be a more significant problem than for women at menopausal age, or postmenopausal. But simply because she no longer wishes to or can no longer bear children is no reason for a woman to unnecessarily subject herself to the possible complications and as yet unknown hazards of hysterectomy. For older women there is no hard scientific data to prove that the womb is totally useless simply because it no longer cradles a developing embryo. Its effects upon hormone production have been noted— there is some clinical evidence that even if the ovaries are left intact, the removal of the uterus appears to affect estrogen production, and patients experience hot flushes and other symptoms of hormonal imbalance.

The operation itself carries with it all the usual hazards of surgical procedures. The first hysterectomy was performed only as recently as 1844. By 1975, in the United States alone, some 787,000 of these operations were being performed annually.[3] Up until about twenty-five years ago, before the availability of antibiotics and life-support systems in well-equipped hospitals, the operation continued to be a difficult and dangerous one, and the tendency was to perform it only when clearly indicated. But today the operation is relatively safe. Nonetheless, surgery carries with it the dangers of pelvic infection, hepatitis, shock, anaesthesia accident, embolism, hemorrhage, and other unwelcome complications.

Fortunately for the woman who really requires a hysterectomy, the operation, performed by a competent surgeon in a well-equipped, accredited hospital, is today a remarkably safe procedure compared with the past. The main problem with it seems to be more the frequency with which it occurs, and the large number of unnecessary operations.

Estimates of unnecessary hysterectomy, from a variety of studies, range from one fifth to one third of those performed. Back in 1941 one of the earliest studies of hysterectomy cases done by Dr. Norman Miller found that one third of these operations in one New York hospital were performed on normal uteri.[4] Later, in an audit of hospital admissions during the 1950s and '60s performed by Dr. Ray S. Trussell and Mildred A. Moorehead of the Columbia University School of Public Health for the Teamsters Union Joint Council 16, Dr. Alan Guttmacher, the famed gynecologist, looking at these data found that one third of the operations were unnecessary and another 10 per cent were of questionable advisability.[5]

In Los Angeles, a team of doctors reporting to Ralph Nader, the consumer advocate in 1971, reported the same rate, one third unnecessary operations.

More recently, in a preventive program, Cornell University Medical College, Department of Public Health, organized a team of surgical consultants in the Greater New York area to provide second opinions before surgery was performed. These services were provided to over 400,000 insured members by various labor unions including the employees of Gimbels and Bloomingdales, the Teamsters Union, Municipal workers, and others. Among those women who voluntarily sought a second opinion before their operations, almost 44 per cent were found not to need them; of those women who were required to have a second opinion by their insurance plans, almost 20 per cent were not confirmed.[6]

The high rate of medically deemed unnecessary hysterectomies is not confined to the United States. A massive study in the Canadian province of Saskatchewan, undertaken in the early 1970s by the Saskatchewan College of Physicians and Surgeons, produced some pretty startling evidence. The College was prompted to do its investigating when between 1964 and 1971 the number of hysterectomies more than doubled—from 1,710 to 2,941, even though the population size had remained the same. This meant that some 633 per 100,000 women in Saskatchewan had this surgery compared with 500 per 100,000, the national average in Canada—an excess of 14 per cent.[7]

The nine-member committee appointed to examine this phenomenal increase in rate—were Saskatchewan women so different from all the others or medical practice so superior or inferior?—were extraordinarily generous to physicians in defining "necessary" operations.

The only operations considered unjustified were those for sterilization, for prophylaxis (preventative treatment just in case something *might* happen), and for age. Yes, in many places, including Saskatchewan, the birthday present for reaching menopause is surgery! This left all the gray areas, including small, benign fibroid tumors as acceptable. Yet, about one quarter were still found to be unnecessary.

There have to be some serious questions raised when the rates of performance of hysterectomy vary so widely.

## Why Hysterectomy?

Not every surgical procedure performed on a woman's reproductive system is the same, nor is surgery performed for the same reasons. It isn't true that every woman at menopause needs a hysterectomy. And there is a distinct possibility that some women who have them do not need them. However, there are women who *must* have surgery for compelling reasons. What are these reasons and what are the surgical procedures that can be expected?

The most clearly indicated reason is that of saving a life. Cancer of the womb, fallopian tubes, ovaries, vagina, or any part of the pelvic area clearly are reasons to perform surgical excision. While in certain situations irradiation, chemotherapy, and the newer technique of cryosurgery (freezing) are used, wherever possible removal of the cancerous growth is an accepted procedure. In these cases, usually, the womb is removed as well as ovaries and fallopian tubes.

But of the over 780,000 hysterectomies performed annually, only 10 to 20 per cent are performed for these and other life-threatening conditions. According to the American Cancer Society, there are only about 67,000 new cases annually of uterine, ovarian, and invasive cervical cancer.

The vast majority of hysterectomies are performed for what is interpreted as disabling conditions due to disease or discomfort in the pelvic area. This covers a wide variety of specific ailments. Among these is uterine prolapse (the dropping of the womb out of its proper position), causing a variety of complaints from discomfort to incapacity for sexual intercourse—there are women in whom the womb drops into the vagina, sometimes protruding from it. Massive fibroid tumors with accompanying hemorrhaging are another problem. In a number of these cases, the womb may be perfectly normal, but, as in severe prolapse, may be causing pelvic congestion or other major discomfort.

## Hysterectomy

In the hysterectomy, the uterus is removed. The usual procedure is for the womb to be removed through an abdominal incision made between the navel and the pubic area. The hospital stay may be up to eight to twelve days. Most women are told they can resume normal and full activity after three months. However, some women find they require many more months—up to a year—before they are as strong as before surgery.

Sometimes the surgeon will remove the uterus and one ovary and the fallopian tube connecting that ovary to the womb. Sometimes a complete *salpingo-oophorectomy* is performed, with both ovaries and fallopian tubes removed.

In younger women, there is a greater tendency to leave one or two ovaries, in the absence of indication of disease, to permit continued hormone production. Sometimes in the case of menopausal or post-menopausal women, the ovaries, even if healthy, are removed as a "preventive" measure. There is considerable controversy concerning whether or not this is necessary, except where uterine cancer is present. Some argue that ovarian cancer is thereby prevented, others argue that healthy ovaries might continue to perform hormone production even past childbearing age, permitting the body to maintain a better internal balance. They maintain there is no need to remove healthy parts of the body.

## Vaginal Hysterectomy

In this operation, the womb is removed through the vagina rather than from the abdomen through an abdominal incision. It might seem to most that this would be a preferable procedure since the abdominal wall is left intact and there is no abdominal scar resulting from the incision. But a hysterectomy is not like childbirth, where the infant normally exits from the vagina, and the Caesarian section, with its resultant abdominal scar, is used only for difficult births. The removal of the womb itself is quite another matter. Abdominal hysterectomy is followed by a period of postoperative recovery which includes time for the abdominal wall and incision to heal. Vaginal hysterectomy eliminates this aspect of recovery. However, while many surgeons consider this procedure safe, easier, and more comfortable for the patient, some studies indicate a higher rate of other postoperative complications which result due to vaginal hysterectomies. These include fevers and urinary tract infections. Scarring of the vagina may also result. Vaginal hysterectomies do not necessarily eliminate any of the other operative and postoperative complications of any major surgical procedure. The choice of method depends upon the particular patient's condition and attitude as well as, most importantly, surgical skill.

## Fibroid Tumors

One of the most frequent reasons that hysterectomies are performed is the presence of fibroid tumors in the uterus. One of the misconceptions that many women have is that if they have fibroid tumors, they require or will require a hysterectomy. This is not necessarily the case, however. Fibroid tumors are lumps of muscle fiber called "myomas." They are benign growths, ordinarily posing no danger to life. However, in about 50 per cent of the women who do have fibroid tumors, there is some menstrual irregularity—pain, cramps, excessive or irregular bleeding, and, in some cases, sterility. It has been estimated that about 500,000 women under thirty in the United States and 50 per cent of all women at the age of forty have one or more fibroid tumors.

In some women, when the symptoms increase in severity they become the reason for a hysterectomy to be performed. Some of these tumors appear to be estrogen dependent for as menopause approaches, and hormonal balance changes, many small myomas shrink or disappear.

There is an alternative to hysterectomy in the case of fibroid tumors, and that is for the tumor alone to be excised. This operation is known as a *myomectomy*. As in the case of most surgery, there are advantages and disadvantages to this operation.

The advantages are the obvious ones of permitting a woman to keep her reproductive organs fairly intact. For those women to whom the womb represents an essential part of their femininity, keeping the womb avoids an assault upon their personality. It thus avoids the psychological disturbance some women feel after hysterectomy.

But there are frequent medical arguments raised against myomectomy. There appears to be greater risk, in this operation, of hemorrhaging. Tumors often grow back. For premenopausal women who wish to have more children, there is the added risk that the fallopian tubes may be damaged, preventing conception. Also, because a portion of the womb may be removed with the tumor, or because of the resultant scarring, there is a danger of rupture of the womb during pregnancy. Of course, hysterectomy completely removes the possibility of childbearing. For the menopausal woman, difficulty of childbearing after myomectomy is certainly not a critical element in a woman and her doctor's choice of operation. Far more significant are the extent of the tumor and the severity of symptoms.

Not all gynecological surgery entails the removal of the uterus or salpingo-oophorectomy. Sometimes only the cervix is surgically removed. In other situations, as described above, a tumor or cyst might be removed, leaving the womb intact. Another operation involves the tightening of the ligaments that support the womb in the abdominal cavity in its proper position between the bladder and the rectum, thus correcting uterine prolapse.

## Dilation and Curettage

Dilation and curettage, commonly called the D and C, refers to the scraping of the endometrium, or lining of the womb. In this procedure, the cervix is dilated permitting the physician to insert a spoonlike instrument which scoops out the lining material. A D and C is performed in the hospital and generally does not require more than one day's stay. It is a rapid and safe procedure when performed in a modern surgical setting. D and C, because it removes the lining of the womb, also removes any pregnancy, and is an abortion procedure as well. However, it is frequently the course of both diagnosis and treatment of many of the symptoms of menopause. Women with highly irregular menstruation, unexplained bleeding, or excessive bleeding, among other reasons, are frequently asked to undergo D and C. Sometimes the procedure itself corrects the condition that has led to the menstrual symptoms. The endometrial material collected is analyzed in the laboratory and the physician can tell whether there are serious pathologies present. Cancer of the endometrium or the presence and extent of non-malignant tumors can be diagnosed. Generally speaking, all women who are advised to have a hysterectomy should first have a scraping of the uterus, and in the absence of cancer, a period of observation and waiting, to determine whether or not the symptoms remain or disappear, should be undertaken prior to the decision to have a hysterectomy.

## Hysterectomy and Sex

Does having had a hysterectomy affect sex desire and sex life? First of all, having had a hysterectomy has no effect whatsoever on a woman's ability to engage in sexual intercourse. In cases where the operation was preceded by severe symptoms such as continuous bleeding, pain, or severe prolapse of the uterus, the ability to perform sexually may even be improved.

What of desire? Is the libido affected in any way? Here the evidence is not so clear—women differ, and their reasons for and reactions to hysterectomy differ as well.

According to Alfred Kinsey, if a uterus is removed, 54 per cent of the women have no change in their sex desire. Some 17 per cent show an increase in desire, whereas 17 per cent show a decrease.[8] Of the 17 per cent who show an increase, it may be that the loss of fear of pregnancy can release inhibitions concerning love-making. Also, some of these women may need to assert their femininity through an increase in sexual activity to prove they are still women. It may, of course, also be that the very illness that prompted the choice of hysterectomy had previously discouraged sex life.

For those who show a decrease in libido, there again may be a variety of reasons. For some women the uterus represents to them the core of their femininity. Its removal and the loss of ability to bear children represent, therefore, the loss of their female nature. In addition to this psychological factor, there are very real anatomical factors involved. With the uterus gone some women sense a loss of feeling, which is not necessarily replaced by a clitoral or more generalized pleasure. Dr. Ken Walker, a gynecologist from Niagara Falls, New York, and author of widely read popular medical books, suggests also that some women use the hysterectomy as an excuse not to engage in sex:

. . . some patients have come to me after the operation and said they no longer enjoyed sex. Well, if they enjoyed sex before their hysterectomy, they'll enjoy it later. I suspect in those cases the women are using the operation as a reason to push their husbands away, something they've wanted to do for years, anyway.[9]

Dr. Walker, who usually cautions against unnecessary hysterectomies, may be right about some of these cases, but it seems that if a woman comes for help because she no longer enjoys sex, it may be precisely because she does *not* wish to push her husband away.

Certainly, there is evidence that for a portion of those women who do undergo hysterectomy there does exist the real possibility that, whether for psychological or anatomical reasons, there is a loss of sex desire. Fortunately, this represents a very small minority, many of whom are likely to be helped with counseling. But the surgery is not without this hazard and should not be undertaken for flippant reasons. There have to be some pretty sober reasons for hysterectomy, such as the existence of cancer or a seriously disabling condition.

## Why Is Hysterectomy So Popular?

There is no single reason why unnecessary hysterectomies are performed, for the many factors that go into a decision by a doctor or a patient to go ahead with the operation are influenced by many things, including medical opinion, fashion, a woman's attitude toward her body, and cultural attitudes in general, as well as, unfortunately, greed. And many arguments can be raised on both sides of the fence in regard to each of these.

Hysterectomy for sterilization is a case in point. Obviously, the removal of the reproductive organs makes pregnancy impossible. A woman, especially in her forties, not wishing any more children and perhaps justifiably annoyed with anxiety-provoking menstrual irregularities, might simply want to "have the whole thing out," have it over and done with. Sterilization by hysterectomy, the so-called "hysterilization" was pretty rare in the United States up until the 1960s. But by the early 1970s the numbers of such operations jumped precipitously. It even received official sanction by the American College of Obstetrics and Gynecology which, in 1971, approved hysterectomy as a method of sterilization. The practice is now growing in Canada as well.

With so many less radical procedures for contraception, such as the

more common mechanical and chemical devices as well as tubal ligation and laproscopy, it becomes increasingly difficult to justify sterilization by hysterectomy. It can no longer be argued that the indi-
gent, the retarded, the incompetent women who are unable to cope
with their bodies, involved in contraceptive failures, abortions, or innocent promiscuity must be sterilized in this radical way. The so-
called "Mississippi appendectomies," the hysterectomies performed
among the very poor women of the South, point to the class angle
involved in such operations. And for women of all social classes who
are both intelligent and competent, the resort to hysterectomy for
sterilization still exposes them to the needless risks inherent in all
major abdominal surgery.

But what of the woman in her forties, approaching or at menopause? She no longer needs her uterus for childbearing. She is likely
to be experiencing menstrual irregularities. She has a fifty-fifty
chance of having some fibroid tumors. She may even be beginning to
experience more frequent episodes of vaginal or urinary tract infection. Do these conditions call for a menopausal birthday present—
the hysterectomy? There are some doctors and many women, too,
who tend to turn to hysterectomy as a matter of course for the middle-aged woman, where some other far less radical treatment would
more easily take care of the trouble.

Women themselves are not without responsibility in the growing
numbers of hysterectomies performed, now that the surgical procedure is regarded as pretty safe. One of the reasons is expectation.
After all, with hundreds of thousands being performed annually, it
isn't hard to imagine that your turn will come, and that it is to be expected—pretty much the way mothers a generation or two ago simply assumed it was normal to have their children's tonsils removed so
they wouldn't get sore throats. I remember the astonishment I felt
when one of my friends, a well-educated, intelligent woman, talked
about the time ". . . when I'll have my hysterectomy." When I
asked if anything were wrong, she said, "No." "Then why speak of
when you'll have your operation?" I asked. "Oh," she said, "my sister
had problems with menopause, she used to be so depressed. I want
to avoid that, so I'll have a hysterectomy."

The notion that hysterectomy solves more problems than it causes
when performed on middle-aged women is very common. But having

a hysterectomy is not so simple as changing the sparkplugs or the battery of a car. The removal of a healthy womb and ovaries, even at middle age or later when childbearing is no longer possible, will not accomplish the solution to other problems a woman might be experiencing in her life which she or her doctor think of as "menopausal."

Canadian gynecologist Ken Walker concurs with the notion that many women think that a hysterectomy is the answer to all their troubles—most of which have little to do with their physical condition. He says:

> More times than I can count, I've had a woman come into my office who's about 45, has three or four kids, and she's got a little pelvic pain. She's also kind of weary with life, worn out, rather unhappy, and she wants a hysterectomy because that's going to tidy up all her problems. But a hysterectomy only cures the immediate physical symptoms. It isn't going to cure too little love, not enough money, and three or four screaming kids.[10]

Obviously, some women anticipate that menopause will carry with it the many symptoms they have learned to expect as the menopause syndrome. And indeed there are many women who, at middle age, *do* experience many problems, even though these are not a direct result of menopause itself. But there are those who have the mistaken notion that a hysterectomy is good for what ails you, whether it be backache, headache, nervousness, fatigue, etc. It has been estimated that as many as 10 per cent of hysterectomies are performed for these complaints, which for the particular women involved had nothing to do with the presence of their wombs, which were healthy. But for some women there is the belief that the womb is the seat of their troubles, and they are willing to pressure their physicians into operating on them.

Dr. Walter Alvarez, for twenty-six years a professor and senior consultant of the Mayo School of Medicine, reports at least one hundred hysterectomies performed to treat migraine headaches without the slightest scientific justification! Frequently the patients themselves demanded the operation in desperation rather than accept the fact of their headaches.[11]

There are also women who have never been comfortable with their bodies, and with menstruation. Attitudes toward the menstrual period as "the curse," and a willingness to put an end to this manifestation of their femininity, predispose them to accept or even request hysterectomy.

Women's attitudes toward both menstruation and menopause are varied. It has been suggested that women's attitudes toward menstruation, for example, can be divided into two clear-cut categories. There are those women who enjoy their menstrual period, who believe that to lose as much blood as possible is good, that it is somehow cleansing, especially if their cultural attitude supports the notion of menstrual discharge as "dirt," rather than understanding its biological function. Some women enjoy the sense of rhythmic cycle they experience monthly, responding to the sense of premenstrual fullness and tension, aware of a sense of "cleansing" and return to the postmenstrual period; some women speak of their feeling "lighter" (at Weight Watchers, many times women will report their weight gains—"It's premenstrual," and proudly point to their postmenstrual weight loss). There is often a sense of good health accompanying a heavy menstrual flow.

Other women, on the other hand, are fearful of menstruation. They are distressed by bleeding, talk seriously about "the curse" as if some evil were likely to befall them during this time, and the sooner done with the better.

Some women are impatient with the menstrual irregularities and flow during the years approaching menopause. Take the case of Mary. At about the age of forty-four, Mary began having unusual, for her, menstrual flows. They were very heavy, often causing her embarrassment as her clothes were stained, sometimes forcing her to give up her usual lively activities as she spent a day or two in bed. Her own physician, when she asked what could be done, suggested a hysterectomy. Mary had several physician friends, one of whom urged her to consult a prominent gynecologist, highly thought of by other doctors. When Mary did, he gave her a thorough physical examination, concluded that there were no pathologies in her case, and that a hysterectomy was not necessary. He suggested the possibility that her menstrual flow would decrease as menopause approached, and that since the operation was not urgent there was time to monitor her condition. But Mary was highly intolerant of the distressful menstruation. She returned to her own doctor and asked for the operation. Fortunately for her the operation was uncomplicated and her recovery relatively uneventful.

But Mary was disappointed in the time it took for her to recover enough strength to be able to lead the active life the periods had interfered with. It took nearly a year before she could resume her normal activities, even though she had thought it would be about three months.

I have always been impressed by the number of women who speak about menstruation as if they cannot wait to be done with it. While certainly this attitude is not synonymous with the desire for surgery to hasten menopause, a woman with this point of view is more likely to report as serious symptoms the very condition that other women consider good and normal. Also, such women are less likely to be distressed by the absence of menstruation, therefore hysterectomy is more acceptable to them.

It is useful to remember the study of Welsh mine women, which found that women with a negative attitude toward menstruation were those women who also had a disturbed conjugal relationship and were making an adjustment to giving up the female sexual and social role.[12] If this is so, then hysterectomy among such women is a dramatic carrying out of this attitude. For many women, the loss of their periods with menopause is fraught with the complex problems of changing sexual and social status.

If these findings concerning significant differences among women concerning their interpretations and attitudes toward the functioning of the womb are true, then physicians are well advised, in the absence of the very real physical, organic indications for hysterectomy— there is no denying that many are in the best interests of the physical well-being of the woman—to make careful evaluation of the patient in terms of her frame of reference. In many instances, the patient's complaints can in themselves mislead; an unbearable flow for one can be that which provides a sense of well-being to another. In the absence of cancer and other serious conditions, these complaints had best be evaluated with the best diagnostic procedures, including a D and C.

Although some doctors are reluctantly pressured by women into performing hysterectomies, even when they do not think them necessary, there are others who are quite willing to go along, especially in the case of middle-aged women. One obvious reason is a medical decision that sees hysterectomy as a means of preventing medical problems in a woman and, since her womb is no longer needed for childbearing, it might as well be out along with the fallopian tubes and ovaries. One of the medical arguments is that with the ovaries removed, some 20 per cent drop in the cancer rate can be predicted. For this reason, women who require surgery for such conditions as prolapse of the womb, fibroid tumors, or who desire sterilization or hysterectomy for other non-life threatening conditions are sometimes advised to have a hysterectomy. The alternate choice of treatment might be, in certain cases, less radical. Other treatments might be irradiation or subtotal operations to repair ligaments, or tubal ligations, cryosurgery, or myomectomy. And, at menopausal age, generally the ovaries are also removed, the medical argument being that since cancer of the ovaries is extremely dangerous and difficult to diagnose, and estrogen production of the ovaries is now declining anyway, the best thing to do at menopause is to have them out. Prevention seems like a pretty seductive argument in favor of radical surgery until you begin to examine its implications. As one critic of this point of view remarked, "You might as well argue that total bilateral mastectomy [removal of the breasts] of all women over thirty-five will reduce breast cancer 100 per cent."[13] Just because the internal organs aren't seen is no reason to be flippant about their removal. And the ovaries do continue hormone production long past menopause. They do count.

Physicians will argue that there are many gray areas in which a medical decision can go one way or another, and while some doctors prefer a conservative course, or watch and wait, others are more willing to take the radical course and operate.

There are other, less palatable reasons for these decisions. The increasing evidence concerning the profitability of hysterectomy. Also, concern about the dominance of the gynecological and obstetrical profession by men, has led some feminists to accuse the profession of male chauvinist attitudes toward women, which lead the doctors to assume paternalistic rights to decision-making about a woman's medical treatment. And, especially in the case of older women, male doctors are accused of carrying out the general cultural attitudes about women's sexual organs not being very important any longer at menopause. It is pretty difficult to prove that a doctor's decision is based on male chauvinism. And having a female physician is no necessary guarantee that she will not also share this general attitude toward the female organs at menopause, or that her medical decisions will be superior—women physicians were in the forefront of such questionable practices as the support for hormone replacement therapy. Probably one way of knowing about one's physician's attitude toward women is his willingness to discuss alternate treatments before surgery as well as his attitude toward the suggestion of getting independent consulting opinion.

## Surgery and Insurance

The many arguments about the high rate of surgery performed in the United States include one that accuses the system originally designed to improve the availability of medical care—the growth of medical insurance plans—as partially at fault. It seems that women who are insured are more likely to have the operation if their plans reimburse the doctor per operation without any peer review by medical committees. With medical insurance available, more women are likely to have this expensive operation, and more doctors willing to perform them.

The facts seem to support this argument. For instance, the rate of performance of hysterectomy in England and Wales, where medical care is provided by the government and physicians' salaries not noticeably larger as a result of the amount of surgery performed, the rate of hysterectomy is less than one half that of the United States. There are also prepaid medical-care plans run by unions and groups, such as the Kaiser Foundation. A case in point would be the Teamster's Union where surgery is monitored, and the rate of hysterectomy is much lower. Also, in those hospitals that carefully audit medical procedures and discourage unnecessary surgery, rates have fallen as much as 50 per cent. When the U. S. Department of Health, Education, and Welfare studied federal employees in prepaid groups—those in which physicians are paid regardless of the anount of service performed—and compared them with fee-for-service plans, such as Blue Cross-Blue Shield it was found that the surgery rates were 44 to 54 per cent higher among the Blue Cross-Blue Shield participants. Clearly, in those insurance plans such as Blue Cross-Blue Shield, where doctors are paid on the basis of the work they do for a patient, the rates of operations performed are much higher. The insurance companies themselves are increasingly concerned about these problems, and in many places Blue Cross-

Blue Shield is now offering its policy holders rights to a second surgical opinion.

This difference in rates has led some people to accuse physicians of performing "hip pocket" hysterectomies—benefiting their pockets rather than their patients. As third-party payers—they are neither the patient nor the doctor—the insurance companies are increasing their insistence on certain standards in the hospitals where surgery is performed and second opinions before they will automatically agree to reimburse a physician or surgeon.

On the other hand, despite the mounting evidence on the inequity related to insurance plans—the variation in rates from place to place —some doctors would argue that the higher rates of hysterectomy do not represent exploitation of insurance plans but rather superior medical care in the form of more not less hysterectomies, and they would argue, for example, that their colleagues in England and Wales do not operate frequently enough.

In any event, now that there is money readily available in insurance to pay for surgery, and the profit motive possibly at work, the old adage *caveat emptor,* let the buyer beware, is well advised. A hysterectomy ordinarily is not considered an emergency procedure. There is time to consider all aspects of the necessity of the case before rushing into surgery. Except in the case of a clearly life-threatening condition, not the reason for most hysterectomies, a few weeks more or less will not make a significant difference.

## When Surgery Is Recommended

What is a woman to do when she reports to her doctor for an examination, whether she has been experiencing some gynecological problem or not, and is told that she requires gynecological surgery?

The first order of business, and perhaps the most difficult to follow, is *don't panic.* Remember, most gynecological operations are not done on an emergency basis. There is ample time to follow the procedure all people should follow in relation to surgery, which is, primarily, to get the best advice possible—to double and even triple check. There are too many (some say up to 2,000,000) unnecessary or questionable operations being performed in general each year.

Dr. Herbert S. Denenberg, a former Pennsylvania Insurance Commissioner, has written A *Shopper's Guide to Surgery* (see Appendix) which provides advice every woman should be familiar with concerning how to avoid unnecessary surgery, and how to get the best surgical care when an operation is found to be necessary.[14] One of the first things to keep in mind is that there is a wide variety of ability among doctors, differences in training and differences in hospital facilities. Medicine is not an absolute science, and you as the patient have a right to consult and consider the alternatives of treatment.

In the advice given by Dr. Denenberg, rule number one is that a person should not go directly to a surgeon for medical treatment, but rather to a general practitioner or internist. In the case of women, this can frequently be a gynecologist of course, but many people feel that women often place their care in the hands of a gynecologist only, when they would be better advised to be examined by an internist as well, for not all medical problems faced by women are gynecological in nature. Why not go to a surgeon directly? Surgeons are pretty important when needed, but after all, their business is surgery and they are likely to be more ready to treat with surgical procedures than others who are more attuned to less radical procedures of treatment. Surgeons are trained to operate. It is their job. They also have to make a living, and there is, according to the American Medical Association's *Archives of Surgery*, a surplus of surgeons in the United States, which means a lot of surgeons are ready, able, and willing to perform.

If you do have surgery, make sure that the surgeon has been certified. In the United States there are the American Specialty Boards which certify a medical specialist after vigorous oral, written, and clinical examinations. There are over fifty thousand Board-certified surgeons in the United States. Osteopathic surgeons may be accredited by the American Osteopathic Board of Surgery. Information on whether or not a surgeon is certified can be obtained from the *Directory of Medical Specialists* found in most well-stocked libraries. It has been estimated that half the surgery in the United States is performed by non-certified surgeons. Some of these are very competent, but it is wise to check according to all the rules discussed here.

Ideally, the surgeon should be further qualified as a Fellow of the American College of Surgeons (FACS). There are about twenty-five thousand surgeons who are Fellows. Membership implies further screening, and the College does stress continuing education.

A patient is further advised that "Even if your family doctor and surgeon agree that surgery is necessary, consider getting an independent consultation or opinion before subjecting yourself to surgery." Consultations reduce operations by as much as 20 to 60 per cent. This isn't simply because your own doctors are incompetent or too quick to profit by surgery. Consultation can improve medical diagnosis and treatment. In a book entitled *How to Avoid Unnecessary Surgery*, Dr. Lawrence P. Williams (a pseudonym) discusses the advantages of consultations:

> The old saying, two heads are better than one, is as true in medicine as anywhere else—possibly even more so, for conscientious doctors have found out that in order to present a problem case to another doctor, they must first review and organize the facts of the case. This in itself makes the problem clearer. A second independent surgeon, moreover, may consider certain aspects of the condition quite differently, throwing a new light on the problem. The chance that other factors pertaining to the surgery will be brought out is greater with a consultation.[15]

In any event, make certain the consulting surgeon is truly independent. One of the ways to make sure he is independent is for him to be told his opinion is sought but that he will not perform the surgery. Also, you can select the consultant, or get a recommendation from your doctor. Some would even suggest you go to another doctor or two for a diagnosis without telling about the first doctor's interpretation. This might conjure up a picture of the neurotic patient going from doctor to doctor, perhaps looking for the answer she wants, some hoping their illness will disappear by definition, postponing needed treatment, others searching for a doctor to operate. Still, there is no question that truly independent analysis might serve to correct an inaccurate judgment made initially and then simply confirmed because of the tendency to go along with the first opinion. Consultation should take place within a short period of time. Delay can be dangerous. It makes a lot more sense to have a medical review team go over your case before surgery than afterward only to find the surgery was unnecessary.

You, as the patient, have a right to request consultation on your case. The ethical rules of the American Medical Association specifically state: "A physician should seek consultation upon request; in doubtful or difficult cases; or whenever it appears that the quality of medical care may be enhanced thereby." No competent, ethical doctor will be disturbed by consultation. Watch out for those who are afraid of another opinion. And there is no need to be forced into a decision without consultation simply because of embarrassment to bring up the subject with your doctor. After all it's your body that is going to be operated on. You have the right to an intelligent, informed, and careful decision, not one based on fear or timidity.

The well-informed woman will probably wish to discuss with her physician, before surgery, why the surgery is needed and the particular procedures he will follow, alternate methods of treatment, as well as the possibility of risks or complications that may occur. There are times, however, when a surgeon cannot be absolutely certain about a condition before surgery. For example, while operating to remove a fibroid tumor only, he might discover ovarian cancer and have then to perform more radical surgery. A patient's consent has to be obtained before surgery—and informed consent is important.

There are, however, many women who prefer to know nothing about their operations and hesitate to question their doctors. Even where labor unions and insurance plans have offered voluntary consultative services to their policy holders, not all take advantage of these provisions.

Curing has always had a strong element of the magical about it, and many people think of doctors as persons very special, above the ordinary, and possessing skills that are beyond the ordinary person's ability to comprehend. It is difficult for many to realize that doctors are human, can err in judgment, and have learned a body of knowledge accessible to all.

Women who prefer to know nothing about their operations and place all faith in their doctor's competence are sometimes in for a rude shock. Roberta tells this story. When the doctor who had delivered her three children advised her, at age forty-six, that she needed a hysterectomy, it never occurred to Roberta to question the suggestion. She had complete trust in this doctor and would have considered it an insult to suggest to him that another doctor be consulted in her case. Her doctor's judgment may very well have been correct, but there is no necessary connection between the emotional or sentimental ties a woman feels for the man (or woman) who helped while giving birth and his (her) skill and competence in judging the necessity of radical surgery at menopause.

Roberta's operation proved routine and there were no complications. Her recovery was uneventful. However, because of her trust,
Roberta removed herself from any responsibility for knowing anything about what was to happen to her. The kindly man who helped
her deliver children was looked at as the paternal figure who would
take care of everything. As a result, Roberta was shocked to discover
that she had undergone a major abdominal surgery, that she now
had an abdominal incision, and that there were months before she
felt strong enough to resume her normal life. Roberta had thought
of hysterectomy as being similar to the times she had had babies,
and consciously or not had sort of assumed the womb would leave
the vagina the way the babies did and that in no time at all she
would feel as strong as ever. She was totally unprepared for the very
different experience of abdominal surgery.

Among the other rules concerning ways of dealing with the surgeon, it is recommended that the fee for surgery be discussed in advance. All other fees as well, including that of the anaesthetist—who
should be chosen carefully either by the patient or his doctor—hospital fees, nursing care requirements, your own physician's fees, and
any other expenses. Any fees that seem to be excessive, such as very
high fees to an assistant or the referring doctor, should be questioned, since "fee-splitting," the unethical practice of giving a kickback from the surgeon to the doctor, sometimes occurs. A discussion
of the fees can serve not only to protect a patient from this practice,
but also can give the patient a better picture of the nature of the surgery to be performed, and the care required after surgery.

It is also a good idea to ask other patients and associates of the
surgeon about him. Of course, popularity with patients and a lovely
bedside manner do not make up for lack of competence in the surgery room. But a long list of complaints by patients who have used
the doctor will not be a good sign. The Directory of Medical Specialists will give you a picture of the surgeon's education and training. If
you have friends or relatives in the medical profession, check with
them about the reputation of the surgeon. It is important that you
have confidence in the surgeon you are using.

Since your own physician, whether gynecologist, internist, or general practitioner, will be taking over your care after surgery, it is important that the doctor and surgeon co-operate and work as a team.
They really should be working as a team even before, in order to

avoid tragic errors. The following story illustrates this point. Jean, while in her early forties, was on birth-control pills. During this time she had surgery to correct a hernia. The operation was uneventful and the hernia corrected. But on the fourth day after surgery she developed an embolism (blood clot) which, if it hadn't been for the rapid skillful care she received in the excellent hospital, might have taken her life. After that her internist kept her off estrogen preparations because of the real possibility that estrogen at her age was related to her developing an embolism. Several years later Jean required a hysterectomy because of massive fibroid tumors. The surgeon, after the surgery, routinely prescribed estrogen replacement. Jean fortunately called her internist who immediately, because of her embolism history, took her off the medication. Her own knowledge may have saved Jean from a real tragedy, but the possibility could have been avoided in the first place had her physician and surgeon worked more closely together on her case.

Considering a surgeon who is part of a group practice is more likely to insure consultation and communication among several specialties and doctors about each case. However, there are all kinds of group practice arrangements, ranging from partnerships, private clinics, to large-scale groups sponsored by labor and management. Sometimes in these groups patients feel that they get passed from doctor to doctor, especially in the larger organizations, or in those that are arranged so that partners can lead the good life. Doctors are entitled to their vacations and some semblance of reasonable orderly hours, but for the patient to find one doctor on his case one day and another on the next visit—according to who happens to be on duty—is somewhat disconcerting. This does not have to be the arrangement, however, and you have the right to know which doctor or doctors are primarily responsible for your care in group practice.

Health Maintenance Organizations (HMOs) are a form of group practice in which the surgeon's payment does not depend on the number of operations he performs. This is different from the usual situation in which a surgeon gets paid according to the number of operations he performs. It has been estimated that HMOs perform up to 50 per cent less surgery than those insurance plans that pay doctors on a per-case basis. In HMOs, doctors get paid for keeping people well, not just for treating them when ill.

A surgeon should also not be so busy that he has no time for the patient because he is rushing from operation to operation. At the same time, a surgeon who operates infrequently isn't the best bet either. To keep up surgical skills, at least several operations per week are generally considered essential.

Modern surgery is not dependent upon the skills of a well-trained surgeon alone. Where the surgery is performed, the facilities of the operating room and skills of the anaesthesiologist and nursing teams, and the postoperative care are major contributing factors in good surgery. Jean's life was saved by the skill of the hospital nursing and medical staff in the absence of her surgeon. The choice of a hospital is highly important. How does one go about making it?

One of the things to keep in mind is that not every doctor is able to practice in every hospital. If there is a particular hospital where you prefer to have your surgery—and that should be an accredited hospital—it is important that your surgeon, and preferably also your physician, have staff privileges there that permit them to perform your needed medical services. An accredited hospital is one that meets the standards to assure quality patient care established by the Joint Commission on Accreditation of Hospitals (JCAH). This organization, formed in 1951, is a joint effort by the American Medical Association, the American Hospital Association, the American College of Physicians, and the American College of Surgeons. Accreditation was initially organized in 1918 to standardize physical facilities in hospitals giving surgical training. Now, however, the Joint Commission has helped to develop procedures to evaluate medical care which became mandatory for accreditation through its Quality of Professional Service Standards adopted in 1974.[16]

No hospital can any longer be accredited without instituting procedures for monitoring the medical care provided within it. The Joint Commission's Quality Resource Center has developed the "Performance Evaluation Procedures for Auditing and Improving Patient Care," a system of medical audit. Now the physician's, surgeon's, and hospital's performances are examined through this kind of medical audit—over time—very different from the days when after getting his degree or board certification there was no defined way of evaluating a physician's performance, and what went on in hospitals remained unexposed. The guidelines of the Commission are designed to identify doctors who are incompetent, careless, or ignorant, and to detect excessive numbers of unnecessary operations or postoperative complications.

The following case illustrates the way in which these quality-control audit procedures help reduce unnecessary surgery. A community hospital in Virginia audited the records of all hysterectomies done there in one year and found that in 31 per cent of the cases there had been nothing wrong with uteri that had been removed. The hospital's Department of Obstetrics and Gynecology then developed more precise criteria for performing hysterectomies. Another audit, one year later, found that the cases in which normal uteri were removed dropped to 16 per cent. These audits are only one way to protect patients and at the same time identify those doctors who appear to be most responsible for unnecessary or poor surgery. In general, an accredited hospital can be expected at the very least, to be conscious of surveillance by the larger medical community. Prescreening surgical patients, by reviewing cases before surgery and including second opinions is another way to protect against unnecessary operations.

Some 5,000 of the nation's 7,200 hospitals are now accredited. Since the Quality of Professional Service Standards of the Joint Commission is relatively new, it is estimated that only 60 per cent of the accredited hospitals are doing their audits properly, but to retain accreditation, all these hospitals will have to institute stringent quality-review programs. Osteopathic hospitals may be accredited by their own group, the American Osteopathic Association, or by the JCAH.

Given all the inevitable hazards of surgery, it is sensible for the patient to be as well-informed as possible in order to make the most careful decision about who will be operating and the hospital in which surgical care takes place. Also, knowing what to expect concerning the nature of the operation and the postoperative care would seem to better prepare the patient, to prevent any unnecessary anxieties. For example, to not know that intravenous feeding is routine after certain surgery could create panic in a patient awakening after anaesthesia to pipes sticking out of her arms. Yet there are some people who would rather know as little as possible, who prefer placing total care and responsibility in the hands of the physicians. For some, faith in God to care for them replaces action on their part. For most people there is no necessary contradiction in their faith in God and their giving a helping hand by checking on their doctors and hospitals.

Because modern medical practice has become so specialized and takes place within large, impersonal hospital settings, the patient as a *person* with *rights* to information, decisions, and care that concerns her is sometimes lost in the shuffle. The medical community has now become more conscious of the need to police itself. Large insurance companies as well as the government are demanding higher standards of practice for the money they spend. Still, the patient cannot always be sure that others will see to it that her interests come first.

Although most physicians and surgeons are ethical, informed patients are better able to insist on their medical rights. But even the best-informed individual is limited within the medical bureaucracy. For this reason advocates of patients' rights argue strongly for representation on hospital boards and other councils to insure a regular program of patients' rights advocacy within hospitals and other medical settings.[17]

Hysterectomy is today a standard and remarkably safe surgical procedure. But like any surgery, it carries with it the risks of unwanted complications from infection, anaesthetic accident, and possible damage to the intestines, bladder, and vagina. There are a number of possible unanticipated psychological postoperative reactions as well. For the woman who needs surgery to save her life or to enable her to live it more comfortably in the face of serious disabling conditions in the pelvic area, the advances of modern medicine give assurances of remarkably safe and comfortable recovery for the overwhelming majority of women.

Given the tremendous increase in the number of hysterectomies performed, however, and for reasons other than the medical disorders requiring this radical approach, it is sensible for women to insist upon knowing the why of this surgery and to get a second independent surgical opinion. As in the case of any other operation, they have a right to question the necessity of the surgery. Once they have determined it is necessary, making certain that the surgery is performed under the best conditions is essential.

# Divorce and Widowhood — on Being Alone

Perhaps nothing is quite as shocking or surprising to friends and relatives as finding that a couple after twenty or thirty years of marriage decide to separate. "Why did this happen now?" they ask. "Didn't they know earlier they didn't want to stay together?" Sometimes the answer is obvious—everybody knew all along that there was trouble and the couple stayed together until the children were grown and off on their own. Sometimes the reasons are not so easily seen.

Middle-aged couples separate for very much the same reasons as do younger ones, with a few other reasons thrown in for good measure. The primary cause is to be found in the fragile nature of the contemporary monogamous relationship itself, the increasing ease with which separation and divorce are obtained, as well as its growing acceptance in the society. The breakdown of religious sanctions against divorce and the glorification of individuality influence the rates. And, for the middle-aged, there is the added pressure of limited time available to experience and live out the fantasies, the new life styles, and the fulfillment of self-interest which are increasingly condoned, even encouraged in the modern world.

Our society is making it easier and easier, often more attractive, for people to be single. Even the national monetary laws sometimes favor the single return over the joint return. Many a widow has found herself living out of wedlock with a man simply because her Social Security check, calculated on the basis of her being a widow of her former husband, would be cut drastically if she remarried. Sometimes welfare assistance is more readily available to the unmarried. Many a divorcee receiving alimony is discouraged from remarrying, because alimony payments would be cut off.

And while it appears that the society values the couple—travel arrangements are always cheaper for two while one pays a penalty for the single accommodations—there are plenty of pressures and incentives in favor of singles. The romantic, glamorous life of the unfettered, always available man or woman is extolled in film and television, in novels, and magazines. The contented couple are simply assumed to be too stodgy, comfortable, and dull to be the content of fantasy and romance. Separation of the married from unmarried in social life is encouraged. In some communities only couples are welcome. But open the pages of any newspaper and look at the ads—dances for singles, theater parties for singles, cocktail parties for singles, tours for singles, trips for singles, hotel weekends for singles, and bars for singles.

It is no longer unfashionable to be single! The newly widowed or divorced have a whole world out there beckoning them to swing. For many, that world looks more inviting from the outside than from within. There are dizzying choices and isolation from the steadying influence of family structures. The unanswered search for the emotional rapport, companionship, trust, and dependability, are not everyone's cup of tea. And the opportunities for transient, sometimes exploitative, relationships force one to be more self-reliant and better able to withstand loneliness than ever.

If singles have their problems, despite the adventure and joy that are held out as the rewards of that state, it is not surprising. Mostly it can be expected because, after all, mankind has had so little experience with the vast numbers of semiautonomous individuals unattached to, not responsible for, and not part of large family structures. For much of the history of the world and in most places, men and women were arranged within social structures—their association with blood relatives (consanguineal kin) and with relatives by arrangement (affinal relatives)—made explicit and necessary according to the traditional codes of behavior. You were either a member of your mother's kinship group (matrilineal descent) or your father's kinship group (patrilineal descent), occasionally both (bilateral descent). Several generations were included in the family, and at marriage women lived with either their own families (matrilocal residence) or their husbands' families (patrilocal residence).

Marriages were arranged between families, and their solidity backed up by the wisdom of older people participating in the choices. Romantic love as we know it was rarely considered a reliable basis for marriage and discouraged for that purpose. Among the Coast Salish Indians of British Columbia, for example, in traditional times, any romantic attachment that overran concern for the propriety of the marriage relationship between two obviously unsuitable partners was termed the result of witchcraft. (We recognize something of this ourselves when we sing "That Old Black Magic.") Far more important reasons for a marriage to be arranged was that the particular relationship of the partners solidified economic bonds and friendship between two family groups; or it may have been that it insured the keeping of wealth or position within the family, as among the royal families of Europe. This was carried to the extreme in Ancient Egypt —Cleopatra was required to marry her brother.

These arrangements did not mean that married men and women did not get along with one another, have deep feelings for one another, enjoy one another. On the contrary, the wishes of young people were often taken into consideration. But the overriding concerns were whether the other conditions necessary for the marriage to work according to the particular values of the society existed. If a woman went to live with her husband's kinsmen, her ability to get on with his mother and sisters in the household was important. If a man went off to his wife's family, ability to get along there was a consideration.

The combinations and variations on the marriage arrangements fill volumes. But stripped down to their essentials, they guaranteed the survival of social groups, they established bonds between groups of people, not just individuals, and they were supported by customs that guaranteed to almost all that they would fit in, with physical support and contributions, and with emotional ties even for those women who had to wait for their own sons to gain high status before they felt secure.

Almost all societies made some provision for divorce, especially in the case of women who were barren or particularly difficult to get along with. Adultery was not a universal reason for divorce—in many societies it was expected, even condoned, so long as the children were known to belong to the family of the married partner.

Marriages everywhere were given public recognition as contractual arrangements by ceremony, exchange of gifts between families, or by dowry and bride price. In the case of the dowry, the bride brought property with her to the marriage, usually in goods, to solidify the marriage bonds; in the case of the bride price, the groom and his family presented the bride and her family with goods. The term bride price is somewhat of a misnomer—the bride is not actually purchased. These customs really functioned to provide a sort of bond to insure that the partners and their families would take the marriage

seriously, for casual dismissal of a spouse—divorce—often meant requirement to return the payment. Things had to get very bad indeed
for a girl to return home to mother, for example, and not be sent
back; or for a man to want badly enough to break up a marriage to
be willing to part with the dowry.

Religious sanctions against divorce, as among Catholics, also serve
to reinforce marital bonds—romantic love seen as too fragile to maintain marital ties without the reinforcement of faith.

In most traditional societies, there were no provisions for single,
unattached adults. Among the ancient Hebrews, for example, there
was no place for bachelors and spinsters. Everyone was expected to
marry and did. Families arranged the matches and left nothing to
chance in this regard. If death occurred, ancient Hebraic law had
specific provisions for the survivors. A widower could marry another,
or he may have already had another wife or concubine—the early
Hebrews were not monogamous. A widow was also encouraged to
remarry. If childless and still able to bear children, she was expected
to marry her husband's brother to bear his heir, a custom known as
levirate. If older, she might live in the home of her grown son (a
surprise to modern Jewish women who find that their mothers often
attach themselves to daughters rather than sons). She could return
to the home of her father. And, if in the rare case she was totally im-
poverished with no relatives to care for her, she could glean in the
fields and vineyards. A divorcee was relatively free. Generally, barrenness was the major cause for divorce. Such a woman regained her
dowry, she was free to remarry, but was not permitted to remarry her
former husband. It was important for him to have progeny.

For most of the experience of humanity with social bonds, marriage, then, has been far more than simply the union of individuals.
Marriage has been part of the social institution of the extended family, helping to establish the bonds that, within particular traditions,
cement relationships and permit the survival of the society and provide for the social welfare of all. The autonomous individual was an
anomaly, fitting in nowhere, relegated to the status of hermit.

The sexual division of labor in much of history made partnership
between men and women useful; and extending the numbers of relatives, rather than complicating life, enhanced its quality, functioning
as social insurance systems, alliances of friendship, and protectors
and teachers of the succeeding generations.

Modern life has replaced much of this with advanced technology and government. An Eskimo man needed a wife to keep his leather garments in good order for the next day's hunting. A New Yorker can trade his wife in for the weekly visit to the launderette. Restaurants do the cooking, foods are prepackaged; the law requires no support of parents, and the wife's mother will look after the children; the state provides schools, and hospitals look after the ill; and fun and sex can be arranged for at the singles bar around the corner. Society devalues the aged and tells us children are superfluous. Wrap all this up in tinsel and gilt, spit it out on stage and screen, and you have a glorification of singleness—denigration of marriage and responsibility. And the nuclear family, fragile as it is, comes tumbling down.

And the nuclear family is fragile indeed, for it is based primarily on the relationship between husband and wife and rests only on mutual agreement arising out of love and companionship. Responsibilities for children, for older parents, religious belief, and tradition as well as the economic dependence of the wife, or at times the husband, will often keep such a marriage intact despite the absence of love and companionship. But remove these, or some of them, and the primary bonds become those of affection. Once these are gone, so is the foundation of the union.

The monogamous, nuclear family marriage relationship places an unusual amount of stress on the people involved. Husbands and wives come to mean a great deal to one another, the volume of interpersonal contact is increased. And while this can lead to new heights of companionship, sharing, affection, and love, it can also multiply the opportunities for hurting one another, being dissatisfied or disappointed in one another. Also, the companionate form of the monogamous relationship, which is expected in our society, while increasing closeness between husband and wife, also creates by that very closeness conditions in which one or the other partner might feel cramped, restrained, even imprisoned by the relationship. Advocates of "open marriage" have argued that the partners in a monogamous relationship need the freedom to develop as individuals outside the bonds of the relationship while retaining primary emotional ties with the wife or husband. But some people are unable to tolerate change, growth, or even privacy in a partner, and thus the strain can grow too great to permit the relationship to continue.

We expect ideally so much of marriage: love, romance, companionship, friendship, fidelity, deep interpersonal response. The village women of Greece sit on their doorsteps passing the evening, while the men gossip and play backgammon with one another at the tavernas and coffee shops. Fewer and fewer modern women, especially among the well-educated, would tolerate a husband's six evenings a week out with the boys. And not only physical presence but deep emotional response and communication is expected between spouses. Their absence can appear as serious deprivation, even cruelty—we have become highly intolerant of anything not approaching the ideal relationship.

Often people do not separate until middle age because other functions and common interests have kept the family together. Children had to be raised and cared for—there are many men and women who feel these responsibilities strongly and maintain the family intact for this purpose. And many people were raised themselves in traditions that did not take marital bonds lightly. Habit and belief are not easily discarded overnight. Embarrassment and shame in relation to one's own parents can inhibit breakups.

With the shift in values—everybody seems to be doing it—and the lessening or absence of responsibility, at middle age the urgency to take the plunge sometimes hits people. It is now or never to live that life one dreamed of; now one is brave enough (or foolhardy enough) to walk out of unsatisfactory, abrasive relationships. Now, earlier inhibitions are gone, and new sexual experiences, new loves, and new lives beckon. Now, perhaps, one is in a better financial position to strike out alone.

Middle-aged women are affected in four ways—they can be left, they can leave, there can be mutual separation, there can be the divorce of their children.

## Being Left

There really is little protection for women in our society, who, after twenty or thirty years of fulfilling in the best way they knew how the role of wife, against being left by their husbands. Poor men may desert their wives. Men with more money, depending upon where they live, may be required to provide alimony or to share property. In some ways these provisions for payment are similar to the customs in other societies, including the ancient Hebrew and Moslem cultures in which the divorced wife was able to keep her dowry. But, except under those conditions of strict religious sanction adhered to by some Catholics, women in modern society must acknowledge the fact that they are vulnerable, no matter what their own behavior or attitude or love. Their years of dedication and devotion to the marriage are no guarantee against rejection. For this to come at the end of their childbearing years is not as great a tragedy as it was in other places and times, when the opportunity for remarriage was nearly absent after menopause. Still, the tragedy of rejection remains. And now, more people than ever are living past the ages when their marriage would, years ago, have been ended by the death of one or the other partner.

Many traditional societies protected women from the insecurity imposed by the possibility of divorce as they reached the end of their childbearing ability. For example, in old China, if a woman had mourned her husband's parents for three years, her husband could not divorce her. Such filial duty and respect shown by a daughter-in-law to her parents-in-law could not be rewarded with abandonment. In addition, if her husband's family became wealthy, she could not be divorced. The traditional Chinese believed that the time of poverty shall not be forgotten. "The wife of the time when we ate the chaff should not be dismissed." What a far cry from the experience of those modern American women who see their husbands through trial and tribulation only to find his money could command a different wife for his new station. And, recognizing the responsibility of kinsmen for the care of people, the traditional Chinese could not divorce a woman if she had no family to take her in.

Divorce, in general, was rare among the traditional Chinese. But this was a mixed blessing. Wealthy men did not discard their older wife. Instead they brought concubines, younger women to act as mistresses, into the home!

For us, divorce has become readily attainable. The legal grounds vary from state to state in the United States and from country to country, but once emotional divorce has occurred, the legal separation is relatively simple to obtain. "Incompatibility," that vague and amorphous term, represents adequate reason in many places, and where the strictures are more complicated, a good lawyer can see that all the requirements of the law are met. In some places we even have a revolutionary concept—no-fault divorce: Florida is one such state which grants this—the partners do not even have to claim incompatibility. As Jessie Bernard, a leading writer on American marriage, points out, "It means in effect that the partners do not really have a lifelong commitment, that the relationship has to last only as long as both partners want it to last. They do not have to prove anything, not even incompatibility."[1]

Now this may be all right for those women who share the sense of values that accords to them the right to divorce as much as to their husbands, and who have entered the marriage state fully cognizant that it will last only as long as each wishes it to. But many women of middle age whose marriages are long standing either never held this point of view or, if they did, believed their relationships secure since they had lasted so long. For such a woman, a rejecting husband leaving at this point in her life is incredible and precipitates her into the need to re-evaluate her whole life and future.

## Women Who Leave

But women too are affected by the headiness that comes with increased freedom from tradition, the breakdown of functions and responsibilities in the family, and a value system that condones hedonism and glorifies the fulfillment of the individual. Middle-aged women, like their husbands, are often confronted with decreased responsibilities for children and a sense of restriction and absence of joy in a marriage. They see the next generation experiencing the freedom from those inhibitions and restraints of tradition that imposed on themselves early marriage and limited sexual experience and required them to play subservient roles. They took on the chores of housekeeping and child raising and furthering their husbands' careers only to find themselves at middle age with energies, desires, and eagerness to explore themselves and the world for a new level of experience. If the husband cannot respond or empathize, cannot tolerate or value growth in his wife, she may find it intolerable to continue the relationship. And sometimes a wife cannot tolerate a husband who demands more of his marriage partner than a traditional housewife. A woman who feels strongly that that is a satisfactory fulfillment of her role, as opposed to the role of the "liberated" woman, may become upset by her husband's disappointment.

Should he become involved with other women seriously or communicate his displeasure in harsh ways, she may decide to leave.

Some women find that after a long marriage they come to the realization that their husbands have become strangers to them. They have grown far apart, have not maintained understanding and open communication between themselves. The young man married because of romantic attachment can look very different twenty-five years later, with the realities of life pressing in. And sometimes a husband's mid-life crises of his own can become intolerable—does he need affairs to affirm his virility? Does he suddenly wish to pull up roots, change jobs, retire, go to new places? Has he become more demanding of attention and resentful of the wife's continuing concern with the children and relatives? Not always is a wife able to give up her accustomed life for the new style sought by a middle-aged husband. It may appear to her that he has become a totally different person, one with whom she no longer cares to be.

A woman too, perhaps even more than a man, experiences the pressures of time. She knows the social prejudice in favor of younger women. If she is to take on lovers, a new husband, a new career, a new education, she cannot afford the luxury of waiting too long. Certainly that old cliché "it is never too late" hits upon a truth; but it does help to have looks, energy, and the time to explore on your side.

Women bring with them to middle age the experience of their own generation, their value system, and the experience of changing values in the present. How they react depends in part on their ability to tolerate change, or the steadfastness with which they hold on to the values of their youth. The only common bonds between women of middle age are their years and the experience of their generation historically—beyond that, they differ in personal experience, social and economic class, ethnic traditions, and resiliency.

Some women find they are a generation caught in the middle. They have valued monogamy, fidelity, and lifelong commitment to marriage, they have grown up respecting their parents and willing to assume obligations for them, they have anticipated closeness with their children and grandchildren. The post-World War II world has experienced social change at an unprecedented rate. Now children go off resenting any obligation to parents; traditional roles change, and the way in which a woman has learned to spend her life—even where she did it very well as wife and mother—finds her devalued for doing only that. She is confronted by seduction on all sides—from the seemingly alluring life of the singles, the careerists, the accomplished. With the years closing in she is tempted to fly off on her own, to relive her life, as it were, in ways impossible given her usual roles. To live it as she believes the next generation is experiencing it, unfettered and free.

In the past, men courteously allowed women the face-saving device of suing for divorce while in reality it was the husband who initiated the actual proceedings. Today more and more women are initiating divorce because *they* wish to leave. A recent poll taken by *McCall's* magazine of its readers, for example, came up with the surprising result that of the 18 per cent of their two thousand respondents who had been through divorce, 64 per cent said that they, the wives, had made the initial decision to have a divorce.[2]

The increase in the numbers of women who initiate divorce is occurring not only in our society but among peoples everywhere in the world where social change is now occurring at a rapid pace. In India, for example, under the ancient Hindu law a woman was required to obey first her father, then her husband, then her sons. A husband could divorce his wife for traditional reasons, such as her inability to get along with his sisters, or barrenness. The extended family of kinsmen was extremely important, and if a wife couldn't fit in, she was replaced.

Before the Hindu Marriage Act was passed in 1954, it was virtually impossible for any of the Hindu women among this 85 per cent of India's population to get a divorce. Now their traditional family form is undergoing change. The family consisting of several generations, each member knowing his appropriate role, is giving way to single-generation families, with the roles of family members uncertain. The Indian sociologist Rama Mehta argues that the change in family form in India has contributed to the rise in incidence of divorce. "As the traditional respect for age and authority was on the decline, the line of authority and responsibility between men and women was no longer clearly delineated."[3]

More and more Hindu women are beginning to institute divorce proceedings—some because they no longer are willing to obey the traditional injunctions to respect age and authority. The increasing numbers of well-educated women, using their influence in society and government and refusing to be subordinates within the family, has resulted in conflicts the women resolve by divorce. Modern Indian women may be facing new trials and difficulties in the unchartered territory of their new lives. Their mothers and mothers-in-law are the generation caught in between, reared to carry on their duties respectfully, finding now that those who come after them do not carry on the tradition.

## Adultery

The Judeo-Christian tradition has taught that adultery is a sin. Thou Shall Not Commit Adultery, as a commandment, has formed the basis of adultery as cause for divorce in the Western tradition. Not all peoples feel this way about extra-marital affairs—often they are ignored so long as the children belong to the legal father. Even with their commandment, the ancient Hebrews took no chances—children derived their Jewish identity from their mothers.

Still, in our society, sexual monopoly by the partners in a marriage is claimed as a right, and infidelity is everywhere a legal ground for divorce. Much of how people *feel* about adultery, however, depends on their expectations of marriage and the social codes they are accustomed to believing.[4] And, the fact of the matter is, despite any of the emotional concomitants of adultery, it is an ever-*decreasing* ground for divorce. Extra-marital relations, on the other hand, seem to be on the increase.

To a woman who entered marriage expecting everlasting emotional closeness with a husband, the fact of his infidelity can be shattering. But many women have been raised to anticipate infidelity in a man. In this culture, extra-marital flirtations are considered feathers in the cap of a man among men. For a wife to engage in the same behavior—that is another matter. The cuckold is considered a fool in fact and fiction. But the old double standard has gone the way of many other social codes. Middle-aged women released from the inhibitions of their youth, affected by the tantalizing dreams sold in the mass media, searching also for fulfillment and enriched experience, have their lovers as well. How this affects their marriages is very varied. Sometimes it means improved sexuality and a new understanding of one's husband; sometimes it reveals major inadequacy and brings to the surface disappointments that cannot be resolved. Sometimes a "fling" is a *divertissement*, a bit of spice added to the regular diet—fun occasionally, but always with the threat of indigestion.

Affairs can be but are not necessarily harmless fun. Humans when they are together sexually, tend also to like to be together—either for a time, physically or, as closeness develops, together emotionally. We fall in love. Our thoughts revolve about the beloved. The mundane, familiar person at home interferes with the dreams. It becomes so easy to find reasons to criticize, to find reasons to stay away with one's lover whether in reality or in fantasy. The necessary deceptions create psychological distance between the partners, forming a chasm sometimes too difficult to breach.

How a woman responds to the knowledge of her husband's extramarital affairs, or how he responds to hers, grows out of a complicated set of values and emotions woven within the marriage relationship. What is perhaps more difficult for some women to withstand is not the fact of the infidelity itself so much as it is the breakdown of trust. Where marriages were not founded on trust, but rather on complex relationships between kinship groups, this may not have mattered so much. But in our time, marriage is primarily founded upon companionate, close relations between a man and woman. Trust is an essential ingredient of such a relationship. Even "open" marriage, in which each partner is encouraged to pursue his or her own individual development, is possible only where the partners find their primary emotional and friendship relationship with the marriage partner. When the chips are down, having made a commitment to marriage, a wife anticipates she is all things to her husband; to accept the possibility of his amours, or for him to accept the possibility of hers, is likely to lead to a head-on collision with the original ideals of mutual trust and exclusiveness brought to the marriage in this society.

Each generation may feel somewhat differently about sexual exclusivity in marriage. Surprisingly, given the sexual revolution of the 1960s, apparently a sexual monopoly is more important to young than to older men and women. This may be precisely because, with greater experience before marriage, young people come to a marriage relationship from a position of conscious choice and commitment, rather than from the need for convenient sexuality and the first flush of romance. This investment of thought and emotion in a marriage carries with it the requirement of closeness and fidelity. Once these are gone, re-evaluation of the relationship becomes necessary.

An occasional romance or sexual adventure need not necessarily change the desire of a couple to stay together. In any event, adultery is decreasingly presented as grounds for divorce. This does not mean that it isn't a factor. Rather, other grounds are now acceptable as well. In our time there is little to keep a couple together except the wish of each partner to stay together. And such a reason is pretty fragile indeed!

Playing musical chairs is no simple solution to marital difficulties. The next relationship is not necessarily any better and may be little different. But we need each other in this difficult world. Being alone is not easy—we seek out a new mate when an old one is gone.

## Getting a Divorce

Divorce is difficult at any age—the emotional, legal, and financial tangles involved in ending a marital relationship cannot help but create trauma and problems for the persons involved, as well as for others associated with them. For the middle-aged woman, however, after an adult lifetime of commitment to a marriage and a partner, the wrenching away from a familiar relationship is even more difficult. Even for those women who have experienced divorce before, or who had few years of emotions invested in a marriage, the change of positions from married to unmarried creates problems for women at middle age somewhat different from those of younger women.

Anthropologist Paul Bohannan, in *The Six Stations of Divorce*, has analyzed the complexity of modern divorce, and the reasons for the painful and puzzling personal experiences which they are for modern Americans.[5] Divorce is extremely complex for there are at least six things happening at once, and these are of different orders and different intensities, affecting people in several different ways. Our society doesn't handle these particularly well—some of them we don't handle at all—as the confusion over rights of grandparents in relation to the children of the divorced illustrates.

The six stations to which Bohannan refers are the emotional divorce, the legal divorce, the economic divorce, the coparental divorce, the community divorce, and the psychic divorce.

The emotional divorce, for at least one partner and often both, precedes the actual breakup of the marriage. Problems of the deteriorating marriage are the paramount concerns of the people involved. There are many reasons for the emotional separation of the partners, but basically what happens is that two people in the process of emotional divorce lose attraction and trust for one another; they withhold emotion from the relationship; they may grow apart in different ways and be intolerant of changes in a partner—rather than responding to growth and change with increased bonds of interdependence and affection, they may become mutually antagonistic. Partners in such a marriage condition begin to feel imprisoned, hating the vestiges of their dependence on their partners, wishing to be free of the relationship. The regard of each partner is no longer reinforced by love for the other. Two people in emotional divorce grate on each other because each is disappointed, feeling cramped and cheated by the partner.

Emotional divorce can occur at any age and may or may not develop into actual divorce. Sometimes the emotional divorce of earlier years does not erupt into legal divorce until middle age when the "now or never" realization hits people: The children now grown, the financial and legal responsibilities lessened, middle-age men and women, often married for twenty years and longer, end their marriages. For some the emotional divorce had preceded by many, many years; the marriage held intact by the overriding concerns of mutual responsibilities.

Emotional divorce can be exceedingly painful. The loss of a partner in this way, the loss of a loved object, is similar in some ways to the experience of grief after the death of a spouse. To be divorced is in many ways worse in our society than is widowhood. As Bohannan points out, ". . . it involves a purposeful and active rejection by another person, who, merely by living, is a daily symbol of the rejection." There can also be profound disappointment at having invested emotional love and affection upon a person unwilling or incapable of responding mutually—disappointment in that person and disappointment in oneself.

For a widow, grief is painful, but society is supportive in that a widow is relatively blameless—she is to be pitied and consoled, she is allowed to express her grief. And there are still the public ceremonials in which friends and relatives appear at funerals and wakes to help the widow over her period of mourning.

The divorcee, on the other hand, is confronted with no such ritualized way of moving from one status to another. She is often considered to blame—what was wrong with her? She is also expected to be merry and socially active.

Reconciliation is possible while a couple are in the throes of emotional divorce. A coming together again, a re-evaluation of the relationship, and a new level of interaction and depth of feeling for one another frequently results. But once the language of separation moves beyond that of personal emotions into the realm of the legal, reconciliation becomes more difficult.

The legal divorce is frequently based on grounds that have little or nothing to do with the actual reasons for separation, but rather meet the requirements of the law. Once the lawyers are called in and the legal papers written, the chances of coming together again grow slimmer. Whole new areas of contention then begin to develop. There is the matter of disposing of and allotting the money and property accumulated by the partners—and any woman who has had to fuss and fume about who gets what and what the financial obligations regarding alimony are knows that if there were no grounds for disagreement before, there are plenty that develop now.

Then there is the matter of the children. Who goes with whom and for how long? It used to be that children were awarded to the custody of the mother fairly automatically. This is no longer the case. Visitation rights are no longer automatic. And with the transiency of people in the jet age, children and divorced fathers or mothers can easily be separated by continents, complicating the whole matter of when and how often one can visit. For middle-aged parents, the likelihood that children are grown probably makes the custody of their own children an academic issue. But middle-aged grandparents face a real problem, as we have seen, in relation to their own children's divorce and the custody of the grandchildren.

In societies where women lived among their kinsmen, especially when they lived in groups in which inheritance was through the female side of the family, divorce could be a relatively simple matter in this regard. For example, when a traditional Hopi woman of the American Southwest wanted a divorce, she simply left her husband's shoes outside the door and he had to go home to his mother. The home stayed in her family, the children were members of her, not his, family. Her brothers were more responsible for their education and upbringing than their father was anyway. She was at home with all the relatives who mattered to her, and aside from the sex and companionship her husband had offered, life was little changed. It was largely her decision to end the marriage when love and companionship were over. Maternal grandparents stayed close to their grandchildren.

But among ourselves, once actual divorce has occurred, there remains the problem of how one is treated and regarded by the rest of society. And here the divorcee begins to face some pretty serious problems. "Friends—they drop you like a hot potato. The exceptions are those real ones you made before marriage, those who are unmarried, and your husband's men friends who want to make a pass at you." Divorce is no longer as stigmatizing an event in the life of a woman as it once was in Western society, but this does not mean that there aren't an inordinate amount of adjustments a woman must make moving into the status of being single.

For one thing, and perhaps the most important, she must now become a whole, complete, and autonomous individual, somebody other than the wife of her "ex." Sociologist Bernice Neugarten has found that single women at middle age and beyond are frequently more satisfied with their lives than are married women. One of the reasons to explain this is that as single women they have to do all of the things which in a marriage one or the other of the couple have been doing. For example, she makes her own friends. Often in a marriage it is the husband who makes the friends the couple sees; or it is the husband who has assumed the role of providing the money or paying the bills, although sometimes the wife does all the checking. More often than not it is the husband whose job has determined where the couple will live. The divorced woman must make these decisions herself in relation to factors other than her marriage.

The woman who was married and now divorced has to assume the chores and to learn all the skills of managing on her own as single women have been doing all along. For some, the tasks are overwhelming, for others, they result in new levels of competency.

The divorced woman must also learn to resolve many questions relative to her relationship with her husband and her own self. Why did I marry? What went wrong? For me? For my husband? Working through the resolution of the many conflicts and new demands of the single state enables some women to reach new understandings of themselves and a new autonomy never before experienced.

## Loneliness

One of the most serious problems confronting the divorced or widowed woman in our society is that of loneliness. We are, essentially, social creatures. Except for those special individuals who go off as hermits and voluntarily disassociate themselves from society like some Sadhus of India, or those nuns and monks who take vows of silence and abdicate from contact with the outside world (although they do live in communities), human beings feel uneasy and even distraught when removed from emotional, social, and physical contact with others. It is as if our very sense of humanity comes to us through the recognition given our existence by the interrelationship we have with people. We could not have survived our infancy without care and nurturance, our values and attitudes are learned from society, and to be too much alone, in the psychic sense, is to remove us from the world of the living.

Divorcees, though perhaps eager to be free of the fetters of an unsatisfactory marriage, and widows, without the accustomed contact with a husband, unsatisfactory and troublesome though he may have been, share with those women who have lost husbands they loved deeply, the need to establish new relationships. They need to fit in, to be clued in, as it were, to a new scene with one actor now missing. And until new ties are established, the emotional loneliness, sometimes even the physical solitude, can be filled with anguish and pain. How paradoxical that on the one hand there is the intense desire on the part of some to be "free," "to be me," and on the other hand there is the retreat from the loneliness that comes with being on one's own.

The scene "out there" may beckon as more exciting, glamorous, and satisfying than the marriage left behind, but it has its share of bad actors as well. And movement into the world of the single is no simple joy ride for most.

It is true that there is a world which Morton Hunt has termed "The World of the Formerly Married," that acts to help divorcees and widows move into a whole new set of relationships with people who

have also been through the ordeals they are now facing.[6] They pass
on the lore about where to go and what to do about legal advice,
where to go and what to do to meet men and women, and, in general, how to go about rearranging their lives now that they no longer
function in the accustomed ways as a "couple."

The physical problems of loneliness are thus less serious than the
emotional problems. There are generally plenty of people about in
the world of the formerly married, in the various social and political
activities, even the bingo games at the churches, to see to it that one
does not have to be physically alone.

Still there is the matter of restriction on activity when there is no
escort. Aside from the social complication, the very real concern for
safety, protection, and company make it difficult for a woman to
move about as freely alone as she could with a husband. As liberated
as we are or would like to be, it helps to have a man by one's side.

To have to shut oneself up in apartments guarded by electronic
equipment, an assortment of locks and barred windows and dogs is
dreadful. It is a price paid for the breakdown of family systems and
life among strangers.

How different from the experience of the women of Kurdistan. A
Scandinavian woman traveling in this region reported: "One of the
strangest things to me was the fact that I never met a Kurdish
woman who thought me enviable. On the contrary: just as they
thought that in my ordinary European summer clothes I was both
poorly and pitiably clad, so they were intensely sorry for me because
I was obliged to travel about the world alone." She wrote that they
would also have ". . . liked to provide me with a large and flattering
escort who would have done for relatives. For that matter, such an
escort was invisibly present when I went travelling alone." A Kurdish
woman travels very safely. "Everyone she meets with knows that her
whole family will come forward and settle accounts if anything
should happen to her."[7]

Still, it is the search for emotional attachments, for the friendship,
trust, and love that provide the security of inner feeling, after the ab-
rasions and trauma of a divorce or widowhood, that are probably the
most difficult of all for modern women.

A woman needs to be able to love and find love. But even if she is
ready, the fact of the matter is that the ratio of available males to females is lower the older she gets. The competition from younger, per-

haps more accomplished women, is more intense the older she gets, and the chances of finding Sir Galahad, or Mr. Right, grow increasingly slim. Indeed, whole new abilities to tolerate what were formerly considered intolerable life styles have to be developed; whole new abilities to tolerate imperfections and differences in people become necessary.

Women who believed in the sanctity and fidelity of the marriage relationship now find themselves searching for and taking lovers; women who, during their marriages, expected fidelity and considered it important, accept their lovers' visits three or four nights a week and ask no questions about their whereabouts at other times; women who believed in the propriety of introductions and male initiative now find themselves accepting blind dates—something they thought belonged to the realm of the teen-ager—or actively seeking out dates, and paying their own way. For the first time women may discover that they really enjoy the company of their female friends—without sex involved—more than they do the company of the troubled, unreliable, and often manipulative men they are now meeting.

For the middle-aged woman to enter into this world of the single requires a whole new evaluation of herself and her standards. And most find the public world of the singles distasteful. They have found that it is their married friends and relatives, who know other singles, who make the safe introductions after all. The world of the matchmaker is still very useful.

The trust and reliability that provide the emotional closeness people need to overcome loneliness arise from a set of shared values, attitudes, and similar experience. Old friends and relatives are among those who are most familiar, who know similar people, who can arrange introductions. This is far less chancy than sharing astrological signs at a singles bar with strangers.

What about sex? Is there any truth to the notion of the merry widow or the gay divorcee? Is the reluctance of married women friends to continue including the newly single woman in the social company of their husbands based on myth or fact?

In our time, at least, the sex revolution has pushed sexuality to the fore in the mass media—it isn't possible to open a newspaper, watch a movie or television, look in a shop window, look at a billboard without the message that sex is in, as if it never was here to stay until now. For the newly divorced or widowed woman, to shut sex out of her life, to turn it off, as it were, is increasingly more difficult and perhaps more unrealistic than ever before. But while society is always more concerned with sex among the young, it has until recently done little to understand the sexual behavior of older people, particularly the older single.

## Divorce-Widowhood and Sex

In an effort to answer questions about the sex lives of widows and divorcees—questions left largely unanswered by the Kinsey Report—sociologist Paul Gebhard interviewed 632 white women between 1939 and 1956, before the so-called sexual revolution opened up the acceptability of sexuality without marriage among many groups for whom this was not openly possible before. Gebhard's findings do seem to substantiate the merry widow, gay divorcee characterizations of formerly married women—at least for those women who resume a sex life outside of marriage. "Once a woman begins postmarital coitus she is extremely likely to have it with more than one man. This generalization applies to both the widowed and divorced."[8]

Gebhard found that the majority of women whose marriages have ended have sex relations while widowed, separated, or divorced. As might be expected, on the average younger women have a higher percentage of those who resume sex relations than do older women. It could be postulated that older widows may have more conservative mores. And, for both widows and divorcees, the older one is the less men there are available.

The recent Hite Report also found that middle-aged women reported on their strong interest in sex and continuing enjoyment. And some also complained of the problem of limited availability of males.[9]

Widows seem to wait a little longer than divorcees before beginning relationships with men—three fourths of the divorcees begin during the first year as compared with about 50 per cent of the widowed. Those women who begin in the first year do so because by then the trauma of the death or divorce has worn off. Also, some women have a stronger motivation to remarry than others, and for these women there was a progressive erosion of sexual inhibition.

While it might be expected that whether one was religious or not, or the particular religion might influence a woman's behavior after the loss of a husband, Gebhard found that it was the degree of devoutness or piety that counted to restrain a woman from re-entering the world of the sexually active, rather than the particular denomination of which she was a part. Also, although in his sample Gebhard found that women past forty had declining opportunities for intercourse—a situation likely to be very different today as divorce rates jump among people past forty and life expectancy is on the constant increase—he did find that their sex experiences were very good, with an incidence of orgasm higher than while married. Why this should be is unanswered, although it might be suggested that different lovers, released inhibitions, and the expertise which increases with age play a part.

## Others Do It Too

There are several societies around the world in which easy divorce is practiced. The accommodations of persons to these systems provide interesting views of how this phenomenon of marital breakup can be dealt with.

One of these societies is that of the North Alaska Eskimo. Actually, Eskimo marriage was hardly identical to the American or companionate patterns. In traditional Eskimo life the family maintained common economic activities, they both produced and consumed their own goods; marriage involved rights to sexual intercourse, a universal feature of marriage; and, different from our ideal companionate marriage, lack of communication between husband and wife was no serious business, although couples liked to enjoy each other's company. Eskimo couples set up relations with other couples who shared friendship, mutual aid and protection, and hospitality privileges with each other. And the so-called Eskimo wife-lending, when it did occur, took place between a man and his Nuliaq, or partner, the man of the couple with whom he and his wife had a mutual arrangement. Sex was not the most important part of these agreements, which constituted a sort of comarriage, but it did occur. Divorce was relatively simple. A man or a woman simply left, breaking the residence bond with the partner. But the marriage could be reactivated at any time the couple decided to live together again, for their relationship was believed to last a lifetime. Thus, Eskimo divorce was more like separation. At one time or another almost all

Eskimos were separated. The practice was exceedingly common.[10]

Reasons for divorce included infidelity, which meant sex outside the acceptable range of persons permitted by the custom of taking a Nuliaq; failure to meet economic obligations; disputes over childrearing, especially when one child was favored by the mother and a different one by the father; personality clashes; in-law trouble; jealousy, barrenness, and other irritations; and leaving for another spouse. Irresponsibility was not encouraged, however, and an Eskimo man or woman who kept changing partners would eventually find it hard to find new ones. An older woman who was divorced or widowed would either have to find a new husband, increasingly difficult at later ages because of the difficulty of survival for the men, or live with her daughter and son-in-law. In traditional times, under very primitive conditions, if such a woman could not be supported by these hardy hunters living under extraordinarily difficult conditions, if she fell ill and could not keep up their nomadic life, such a woman would voluntarily stay behind, to die alone on the ice. There simply was no room for the ill and infirm.

The Eskimo experience with easy divorce seems to parallel the experience in modern life. As divorce becomes more accessible, so do people in marriage expect their partners to live up to the ideals of the marriage relationship. If they don't, the marriage is likely to come apart. In effect, this forces people to be responsible for their behavior within a marriage or else it be ended. The difference between us and the Eskimo is the kind of behavior, the ideal to which we aspire and which we anticipate.

For our marriage to work, to last, requires an inordinate amount of sensitivity and response of partners to one another, and recognition of the dangers of behavior that fall outside the ideals we expect. That's a pretty difficult recipe to follow, and often the cake falls flat. Divorce for us is so often a painful, distressing condition, compared with the relatively casual Eskimo, because with all of its problems, we have been expected to maintain marriage ties, to constrain the disagreements. This may be changing, however, as social values that condone hedonism, demand constant happiness, and condone the thinking of one's self as primary, take hold in the society. The anguish, sleepless nights, and the soul searching that precede separation in our society may be more the case for middle-aged persons raised on earlier standards and values, which saw personal responsibility for the success of a marriage. Now, if things are even a little less than perfect, they become intolerable. And with one no longer being in the vanguard of the movement—after all, one third of marriages end in divorce, and that doesn't count the number of desertions and mutual separations—it no longer seems so strange to give up one relationship in search of another or perhaps none at all.

It was far more traumatic an experience for an Eskimo to break up with his parents or his brothers and sisters than it was for him to separate from his wife. In our culture it seems we owe increasingly little allegiance to any of these relations.

The Kanuri of Bornu Province, northeastern Nigeria, are another people who experience separation equivalent to our divorce in a large percentage of their marriages.[11] These are a people who practice polygyny, a husband can take several wives. The most highly valued women are young virgins. They are valued not so much for their sexuality—the Kanuri recognize that older, more experienced women are more desirable sex partners; it is rather that young virgins require the payment of a higher bride price by a man to her family. Thus, being able to afford such a bride is symbolic of a man's high economic position, just as young women are status symbols to wealthy older men in our own culture. The Kanuri admired a man who could afford his own plaything—a woman no other man had known.

Generally, men cannot afford such wives until they are older, thus girls marry men thirty to fifty years older than themselves because only these can afford to marry them. Although 45 to 55 per cent of the marriages end in divorce by the fourth year of marriage, after a ninety-day waiting period the women could remarry, and they did. As a woman grows older, her value decreases until by the age of forty-five or fifty she is no longer considered marriageable, primarily because her role as childbearer is nearly over or over.

These are an Islamic people; male dominance is strong. Divorce is very easy. A wife could be divorced simply because she did something her husband didn't like, such as going out of the secluded women's quarters to buy something from a vendor in the street. Divorce itself was easy; a woman could be divorced on the spot simply by her husband stating, "I divorce you," three times.

Being a divorcee was not necessarily unattractive to a Kanuri woman. She was liberated in many respects, able to move more freely and with fewer restrictions than when married. She could take lovers, she could visit about freely. Curiously similar to conditions now common in our own society, it has been observed that ". . . the lack of restraint of the divorced status and the excitement it offers is always there as a stimulant to any marital conflict."

Long-term marriages were rare, but women remarried frequently. But what happened as the women grew older? For one thing, younger wives were brought into the household. This was not necessarily a disadvantage in that sometimes a husband turned over money for management to the senior wife who then had much authority among the women. Also, some women, because of the great skill at diplomacy and their intelligence, retained privileged positions in the household and were not divorced.

Kanuri women knew that with increasing age, generally, their futures were precarious and they did several things to insure against the vicissitudes of middle and later age. For one thing, some managed to make themselves indispensable adjuncts to their husbands, becoming their chief subordinates or *wakil*, in effect taking on a governing role usually open only to men. This required a high order of diplomatic skill and a high order of intelligence. Not all women were able to achieve this high status.

The other thing a woman did was to take a high interest in the inheritance potential of her own children as opposed to the children of her husband's other wives. This, of course, increased tension among wives, but at menopause, when a woman generally left her husband, she could live with her son or sons—having made sure they received their proper inheritance guaranteed for her so she would live comfortably at that time. She might also return to her family to live with her brothers who were responsible for her. And she had one other trick up her sleeve—if she had in the course of her several marriages married a rich man, she might return to his household to be cared for. In general, men feel a strong obligation as well as expectation that they will look after their mothers in later life. For a woman to be concerned about the well-being of her son is considered normal. No "Jewish mother" jokes in such a society.

## Making It Alone

It is perhaps cynical for modern women to expect, on the whole, that more and more women at middle age can expect to be divorced.

In the past widowhood was an unwelcome fact of life. Now that life expectancy for men as well as women is increasing, widowhood is frequently replaced by divorce.

If there is any lesson to be learned from the experience of the Kanuri women, different as their society is, it is that preparation for this eventuality may help buffer the dangers of being alone, whether because of abandonment or by choice. So long as we continue to share the expectation of emotional closeness and fulfillment in marriage, divorce will continue to bring pain and anguish. But by not providing in some way for women alone in their later years, we have an unsatisfactory state of confusion. And there are limited solutions in our society.

Unlike Kanuri sons, our children are not obligated by law or changing custom to expect to or be required to take a single mother into their household, or even to support them. And fewer and fewer modern women care to live with their grown children anyway. We don't even provide the physical facilities for this to happen. Look at the new, modern apartment buildings in the cities and count the numbers of "studios"—room for one and an occasional visitor to share a bed. Hardly the place for one's mother. And daughters-in-law, unlike the biblical Ruth, are not ordinarily expected to bow to the dominant mother-in-law according to the rules of filial piety and respect. Indeed, mother-in-law is seen instead as meddling and unwanted, and the more distant the relationship, the safer her own marriage.

In reality, of course, while not obligated to do so, sons and daughters do help older parents who require financial assistance. However, we do not necessarily value this, either as parents or as the children. These are irksome responsibilities, especially for the greater majority of people living in nuclear families barely making it on their own. Women in traditional families, as among American Indians and working-class blacks, are less cut off from the obligations of willing and affectionate support from succeeding generations than are middle-class women, whose children value lives independent of their relatives.

As far as who will support a woman after a divorce or widowhood is concerned, the trends in modern society are pretty clear. More and more women are supporting themselves, depending less on alimony than ever before. In this respect divorced women are little different from married women, the majority of whom are working as well. Women in the United States now spend an average of over twenty-five years in the labor force compared with an average of eleven years at the turn of the century.

The fact that most women, even with financial assistance of ex-husbands, must return to or enter into the labor force to maintain themselves financially, affects middle-aged women in several ways. Those women who had devoted their energies and talents to childrearing and support of their husband's role in society may find, when divorced at middle age, that they have not developed themselves either by education or experience for work at the higher levels. They may have to undergo "retreading," or retooling, in order to take on jobs that are both interesting and supportive. They may have to return to school—a long and tedious experience at this point in life for some, but exhilarating for others. They may have to develop commercial skills. They have to compete with younger women and men for positions. They may discover new capacities in themselves they never suspected existed. Both physical and psychic energy are needed to contend with the new demands for self-support.

For the woman who has always been in the labor force, to be now dependent on herself rather than having the resources of a shared unit—husband and wife—introduces new anxieties and responsibilities for self-support. Most women in the United States are neither as well paid as men nor in the higher economic positions. To make it on one's own is even more difficult for women than it is for men—and it is difficult for men as well—in our society.

And again, the divorce of a daughter particularly brings to the middle-aged woman, divorced or not, the added responsibilities for the financial aid for that daughter and her children when the ex-son-in-law's contribution remains low or nil.

Unlike so many other societies in the world, and other times, the divorced or widowed woman has few kinsmen on whom to fall back. Most divorced people maintain their own households and do not live with relatives. The spinster aunt living with the family seems a thing of the past. Single persons, in general, maintain their own homes.

With the rise of no-fault divorce and the pressures toward equal rights, it is likely that in the future alimony may not be as available to cushion the financial blow that comes to a woman when the man who has supported her, as is often the case, for many years, now cuts the bonds. If a man is very rich and considerate, he may of course bestow enough money on an ex-wife to see her through the years—much the way Muslim men provided for their older wives. But once the sanction of law is removed in this regard, a woman cannot actually be certain that this is going to be the case.

Essentially, more and more women at this age are required to fall back on their own resources—cynical as it sounds, they must be prepared to look after themselves. There is a price that is paid for the freedom of modern life and modern marriages based not on the wishes and considerations of extended families. Our movement away from dependence and mutual support among relatives toward a glorification of the individual and his freedom from an extended family structure includes the need for that individual to stand on his own. While we need others for emotional support and to contend with loneliness, there are few to fall back upon for financial dependence. If we are really in trouble, there is always the state. Social Security, minimal as it is, has replaced the support of kinsmen; insurance funds, hospital care, professional entertainment, and friends made at work or play have replaced the systems evolved throughout history to protect and support people.

More and more women, then, are required, unless they are able to manage a quick remarriage or liaison with a man willing to support them in their former role of dependent wife, to support themselves. A woman who has devoted all her energies and talents to her family may not be as well prepared as a woman who by education and experience has maintained contact with a world outside the home. Job skills, careers, are some of the things that a woman needs to increase her self-sufficiency, in the absence of the automatic filial piety that insured her care in the past. Her relations with modern children are likely to be vastly improved precisely because of her interest as a person outside of the traditional mother and wife roles once she has reached middle age.

In recent years investment companies and banks have been appealing to women. Their ads run something like this, "When John was alive he took care of all the money. I didn't know a thing. Now that he's gone I turn to the Friendly —— Corporation. They handle everything so well." Well, women who "don't know a thing" about their family finances are probably a figment of the imagination. They may not know everything, but certainly women are generally involved in the management of money, even if it be only the household expenses, and they generally have an idea of how much their husbands earn. They know how much they themselves earn. The picture of the ignorant, incompetent, adorable little woman is a disservice to women in general. There are such women, but they hardly represent their sex.

What is true, however, is that often in marriages women have no property or money in their own names, or even in joint accounts with their husbands. And in these cases, at times of divorce a woman can find herself financially stranded, having been totally dependent on her husband. This is a curious situation in the modern world—the eventuality of divorce in many societies has led people to devise customs to protect women in this regard. Moslems and Hebrews allowed women to keep their dowries; bride price was often returned; even in contemporary Greece where there is a dowry custom still, the law states that if the dowry has not been signed over to the husband, which is not the usual case, at divorce the woman retains rights to that dowry and can take it with her.

In the United States, women retain rights under their husband's Social Security if the marriage has lasted twenty years. But in 1976 the Supreme Court ruled that women with dependent children lose their rights to Social Security (under their husband's coverage) if divorced before that time. The state has clearly not completely filled the void left by changes in the family.

We still have the custom of alimony, but that is gradually being replaced. Community property laws in some states protect dependent women in that the property the couple has accumulated must be equally divided. No-fault divorce makes a woman most vulnerable— she may be given some support for the initial years after a divorce, but not for her lifetime. It seems that the most protective procedure for a woman is to keep some money or properties in her own name. There is little excuse for not being knowledgeable about the mundane problems and tasks surrounding money and its management. There are really no mysterious secrets in keeping accounts.

Fortunately, in our society, a woman is valued for qualities other than her ability to bear children. With one third of her life stretching before her, women at middle age, whether divorced or widowed, are not cut off from remarriage, if that is what they wish. We are not boxed into those traditional customs that run the gamut from the extreme of burying a widow along with her deceased spouse to hurrying her off to sons or brothers.

But remarriage is not that simple. For one thing, the numbers of available men are limited. I recall being told by a Russian woman of fifty that she was unable to live in Moscow because she had no residence permit. Her husband, along with 18,000,000 other Russians of her generation had been killed in World War II. She said she would be permitted to live there if she married a Moscow resident. "But that would mean taking a man away from his wife. I wouldn't do that. But," she added, "many women do."

The experience of the women of the Caucasus is heartening; many of them marry for the first time in their fifties and sixties, their femininity, sexuality, and marriageability extending throughout their lives. And among ourselves, despite the handicap of a skewed sex ratio, older women can and do remarry if they wish.

Divorcees remarry despite the problems of earlier marriages. These relationships are probably not as innocent or naïve as earlier ones— like the ad that says, "The last man I trusted was my first husband." Often they are better relationships than existed in the unsatisfactory marriage. Mature people have learned to be good to each other.

Widows sometimes find remarriage difficult, yet throughout the history of society, there has been much more experience dealing with the problems of widows than that of divorcees in later life. With life expectancy increasing, both for men and women, and with the divorce rate increasing at the later ages, we are beginning to realize the unchartered territory into which the single, formerly married, older adult is being thrust. How to readjust to this new status is fraught with difficulty.

As in all transitional states, the first step is complete separation from the previous status. For the widowed there is much greater social support in this regard. All societies provide for some separation of the dead from the living—if we except that rare matter of widow burial. Funerals, religious ceremonials, proscribed periods of mourning, expected expressions of grief—these required rituals all serve to see the departed off into another existence, and to leave the living free to go on in this one.

The memories of the deceased, the guilt in relation to the things undone or unsaid while they were living, the mixed emotions about being the one left alive, the fear of loneliness, the fear of death so close, are allowed their expressions in tears, wailing, periods of isolation, abstinence, clothes-rending—any of the myriad of different customs around the world. Sometimes the danger of the memories and the continuing influence of the deceased are expressed as fear of ghosts—spirits that have to be mollified or sent on their way not to hover about and disturb one. How does a divorcee rid herself of the impact, memory, or even sight of her living ex-husband? His presence is potentially constant. And we have no ceremonials beyond a perfunctory divorce party to speed his ghost on his way.

The mourning widow is permitted her grief, her allotted time for healing the wounds of a marriage torn asunder. The divorcee has no such approval for the anguish and pain suffered through both emotional and physical divorce. People around may wish to empathize, give solace, but with no ritualized traditional system to help in the process.

In traditional societies a widow knows what she must do. Often she must dispose of the property of her deceased husband, give it all away, or burn it. She must leave for a new place to live. Two functions of these customs are obvious. The fear of evil spirits, or disease as we might term it, prompts the removal from the goods and home as a sanitary precaution. But more often than not, this is not the reason. Rather, it is an understanding that separation is necessary for a life to continue for a widow. One analysis of death customs among seventy-eight societies around the world found that widows and widowers were more likely to remarry in societies whose customs encouraged breaking ties with a deceased spouse, for the breaking of these ties both eliminated memories of the deceased and encouraged psychological distance from him. The researchers found a significant connection between the existence of tie-breaking ceremonies and the percentage of widows who marry one of their deceased husband's relatives or clansmen.[12] It is as if, with a husband waiting in the wings and social pressure to remarry, the culture takes no chances on permitting the deceased husband to interfere with the woman's readiness to take on a new life, and the woman is pressured into removing herself from attachment to the deceased spouse. Traditional Jews practice tie-breaking ceremonies. The deceased is rapidly buried, and there are prayers and a brief period of intense mourning. Clothes and belongings are disposed of soon after the death and widows moved to new housing. A final ceremony one year later frees the widow to remarry.

Translated to our time and society, it might be suggested that more widows and widowers would remarry if they were encouraged to dispose of the goods of the deceased and to move to a new home. But many aspects of our culture interfere with this.

One of the things that sometimes interferes with the readiness of the widow to remarry is the sense of fidelity to the deceased husband. For those women who hold deep attachment to the notion of lifelong monogamy, to take another husband is tantamount to breaking the marriage vow. Several years ago, in that hit Broadway musical *The Land of Milk and Honey*, the middle-aged, widowed heroine, played on the stage by that incomparable lady, Molly Picon, unexpectedly met a gentleman who courted her and asked her hand in marriage. In a charming expression of this notion of fidelity the star turned her face upwards to the heavens and addressed her dearly departed: "Please, do you know what it is to go to the butcher to buy lamb chops for one?" and, "Please, I need someone to bring a glass of water in the middle of the night." Needless to say, she felt the permission to be granted.

These attitudes appear in other places and times as well. In parts of old China, widows were expected to remain faithful to their husbands after his death. And the roads and streets of old China held monuments to these faithful widows. Divorcees have no such necessary or expected loyalty to divorced husbands. But "the memory lingers on," and there are limited aids to making a complete break.

Also, there is a tendency for us to consider the disposal of goods and picking up and leaving for a new life or place as rather frivolous and foolhardy. The assistance of such actions in achieving psychological distance from the departed should not be underestimated. But unless there really is something out there waiting to claim the newly single woman for remarriage or a new, full life, she risks being out in limbo. It is difficult to give up the mementos of a lifetime together. Acquiring housing, making new friends, adjusting to new environments, represent unchartered terrain. There are few brothers-in-law out there ready to take over as they did for the traditional Hebrew women.

Many women may find, if they are fortunate enough not to be

widowed, that with the middle years new joys and pleasures, new degrees of tolerance and understanding become possible within their marriages. The enticement of the single life becomes less seductive the more one sees the trials and tribulations of those caught in the web of the amorphous, experimental transition between being married and other than just divorced.

Where are we heading? It is presumptuous to do more than offer the possibilities. For some, at middle age a new re-evaluation of life will lead to a more satisfactory marital relationship based upon trust and the confidence that years of experience have provided. For some, the traumas of the marriage are too great, and divorce results. Others are widowed. Now the life of being single in ways scarcely experienced before in the history of mankind must be faced. This may very well thrust women into levels of competency, friendship, and sharing with others unknown before in their lives. And the widowed are likely, except those still practicing traditional life ways, to find much company among the divorced. To be married or unmarried, hopefully, will not compete with each other for ascendancy as the life style. No one way has ever been satisfactory to all, and social isolation of the different groups can only lead to the sense that one is missing something by not being on the other side.

# Growing Older Is in Style

Menopause is a universal fact of life for the human species. But never before in the history of the world have so many women lived long enough to look forward to over a quarter century of life after the close of their childbearing years. With the life expectancy of women climbing above seventy-five, the potential for prolonged and active participation in sexual, social, and economic life has become reality long past the years of traditional contributions women have made as mothers, wives, and as workers.

While the physiology of menopause is now better understood than ever, far more medical research and serious attention to the occasional problems faced by a minority of women is required. But the overwhelming evidence points to menopause as a normal, trouble-free culmination of changes in hormonal production in the body, requiring only limited intervention for carefully diagnosed conditions. Attempts to treat a whole generation with estrogen replacement thereapy, now discredited, fall within the category of all the illusive searches for fountains of youth, the waters more often tainted than not. Menopause is not a disease, it need not be disabling—indeed, can even be emancipating from concern about childbearing at a time in life when having children is neither desired nor particularly wise.

Neither need the middle years present, inevitably, extraordinary social and emotional problems for women. They need not, but they often do, for in many places and at many times women have been valued primarily for their reproductive capacity, although their value as contributors to the economic life of the group was also high. Dynamic, modern industrial society has prolonged our lives but hasn't as yet figured out how to provide a gracious environment for our aging population. The young, hopefully, will continue to reproduce. But the species is no longer threatened primarily by the dangers of extinction through no reproduction, as might have been in the ancient past. We are far more threatened by overexploitation of the planet's resources, the potential destruction with lethal weapons, as well as the absence of gracious living and fulfillment as life expectancy increases.

Women, in the experience of societies around the world, have demonstrated their capacity for full, happy lives during and after the middle years. They have been leaders, fulfilled important roles, and, despite the disbelief of youth-oriented Westerners, have continued to be sexually attractive, desirable, and active.

Inability to reproduce is no longer the barrier to social value that it once was. And the modern world opens more choice, more excitement, and more potential for living fully no matter what our ages.

Unfortunately, unless there is a marked breakthrough in the survival rates of men, women of middle age can look forward to the prospect of large numbers of themselves approaching old age as widows. In the United States there are sixty-nine men for every one hundred women over sixty-five, and predictions are that by the year 2000, there will be sixty-five men for every one hundred women. And, as one Census Bureau official states, "The world of 2000 will have a population of fairly sophisticated, educated, elderly women, many who had outside work and have held managerial and professional positions."[1]

Being well educated and having a high income and occupational level is on the side of living longer. As we've seen, today's women, approaching middle age and already middle-aged can, on the whole, expect some twenty-five to thirty-five years of life beyond menopause. Retirement from active life is hardly necessary. Despair is wasteful of energies. A forthright confrontation with the chance to live out one's life from the considered vantage point of the maturity of mid-life is a glorious opportunity. Being a modern woman in the modern industrial world provides alternatives never before available to women on such a large scale—the choices are there to be grasped. And older women will not be alone. As our century nears its close, even the population aged seventy-five and older will have grown at two-and-a-half times the rate of the population as a whole. And those over sixty-five will have jumped from a little over 10 per cent of the total toward 17 per cent.

It will be increasingly fashionable to be middle-aged, as the infants of the post-World War II baby boom reach their forties in the 1980s.

The problem of 1980 may turn out to be quite different from the Orwellian fears of an automated future. The more serious issues will revolve about our growing tendency toward early retirement—most Social Security applicants are now under sixty-five, and who will support both that and other pension systems so dependent upon the contributions of younger workers. With all our sophistication about population control and individual freedom and fulfillment, society may have to return to the ancient wisdom about rearing a new generation for the protection and care of those who came before. With a trend toward an older population, it may be that society will find it necessary to increase opportunity for the middle-aged and older to work and continue in positions of responsibility in contrast to our past attitudes of demeaning the old.

Roles for women are shifting everywhere. Women are being exposed, together with others, to the effects of industrialization and modernization. And never before in the history of the world have middle-aged women been as caught in the generation in between— reared to respect traditional values that more often than not served to control the behavior of adult children, themselves. They were subject to the requirements imposed upon them by their parents. They were raised to respect those values that permitted the old ways to continue. But their own children are the products of experiences markedly different from those many of their parents sustained. Their children, everywhere in the world, are carried along in the inexorable movement to the cities, to jobs and careers outside the home, sometimes across continents to contacts with ideas and people unrecognizable to their parents and grandparents.

This is not a new phenomenon, certainly. It has happened at other times and places for one generation or another throughout history as cultures change, as new lives replace the old. But since World War II, the acceleration of this change is more marked than ever. To the children of the American immigrants who arrived in the early years of this century, their sense of generational change, their being caught in the middle is sharp. They know they were raised to care for their parents, to respect tradition, but they and now their children have been confronted with new demands for their time, their energies, and their belief. Their own children seem no longer to carry on the traditional conservative ways and have dispersed throughout the land, with new ideas and life styles that boggle the mind.

But this experience is not peculiar to this group alone. Throughout the world, in the developing nations, the shift from the land to the cities, from the old ways to the new, goes on.

Middle-aged women experience modernization in many ways. So much of how they are affected or how they respond to the pressures of a changing world depends upon their degree of formal education in the schools increasingly available in all the new nations. The more education, the more potential options in life style open to women. Even in the United States universal schooling existed for little more than one hundred years, and only since World War II have most young people stayed in school through the high school years. In many areas of the world, only since the 1960s has national primary schooling become available to all, and there are many places where it still does not exist.

Work now moves outside the home in new systems of production, removing the traditional patterns of family life, separating mother from child and wife from husband in modern methods of production —something Western women have known for centuries, but now affecting women in remote areas of the world as well.

For a woman to have become modern before reaching middle age may present a different preparation for aging than for a woman to have lived a traditional life—only to find her own children experiencing totally different conceptions of what life should be like. A woman with modern education and experience can grow along with the next generation—her training prepares her for change. For a traditional woman, the break can be, but is not necessarily, traumatic. Traditional women can be very supportive of the young as they prepare for life in a changing world.

Alex Inkeles and David H. Smith have examined the characteristics they believe describe the modern individual as opposed to the traditional, in their book, *Becoming Modern, Individual Change in Six Developing Countries*.[2] Their description seems familiar to members of the modern societies of the world, where most people seem to have these characteristics. Modernity is characterized by openness to new experience, contrasted with the more closed systems of those societies that limit experience to the traditional or known. Modern men and women are ready for social change and willing to accept it. There is the growth of opinion. People are increasingly disposed to form or hold opinions on a wide variety of issues. In addition, people in the modern world are aware of the diversity of attitudes and opinions around issues, even valuing variations in points of view—different from the automatic assumptions about the rights or wrongs of issues characterizing the more closed systems of traditional societies; modern people actively acquire facts and information. Modern man is concerned about the present and the future more than about the past. He believes he can exert considerable control over the environment—fatalism and predestination play a smaller influence. Planning over the long term, both in public affairs and private lives, is believed possible. And that ability to plan is supported by the notion of calculability of trusts—that the world can be understood and figured out, that people and institutions will meet their obligations. It might be added that if they don't, they can be held accountable.

Modern life is characterized by high valuation placed upon technical skill, on justice not based on whim. Aspiration for both educational and occupational levels are high. There is an awareness of and respect for the dignity of others and an understanding of modern production.

If this sounds like a description of the well-educated, industrial Western individual, it is because, after all, it is precisely they who are modern. Whether modernization will take on the same forms and characteristics everywhere in the world is difficult to say—it is likely that particular social traditions and customs will lend themselves to variations on the theme. But in general, modern industrial nations tend to produce people who function in this mold.

Modern people tend to be informed, participating citizens of national states rather than only members of family groups. They have a marked sense of personal efficacy. They are highly autonomous in their relations to traditional sources of influence, especially in personal affairs. In other words, they stand apart from the traditional expectations and influences and are more willing, even insistent, to set out on their own, making their own personal decisions about the course of their lives. They are ready for new experiences and new ideas—open-minded and relatively flexible.

While, again, these characteristics might be said to describe modern Western industrial bureaucratic society and may not apply to all people equally, the fact remains that as nations acquire modern industrial, political, and educational institutions, more people begin to function in these ways.

Many questions remain concerning the course of modernization. Is it inevitable and irreversible? For example, as workers move from less-developed areas to the modern urban centers—as did the people from rural Italy, Greece, Spain, and Portugal to Berlin, Hamburg, and other major centers of northern Europe—on their return do they go back to the old way or bring with them the lesson of modern life? Is modernization a lifelong process or are there plateaus, does it end at thirty-five or forty, when mid-life begins to set in? These are not simple questions to answer, and probably no one answer fits all persons anyway.

Sometimes people move back and forth between modern traditions and folk traditions, with what appears to be minimal strain. With the jet age whole families move back and forth from rural Greece to New York City, from Puerto Rico to the mainland. West African youths move back and forth between European universities and tribal homelands.[3] Middle-aged women are "modern" with their daughters, "traditional" with their mothers.

Sometimes people experience one way of life for a period of years and another at a different time.

British anthropologist Kenneth Little, for example, studied African women in towns, observing many of the changes that are occurring for women as a result of modernization.[4] These women start out at an educational disadvantage to men. They are confronted with new values that stress individualism versus the communal life styles practiced by the large extended families in the countryside. In modern towns the new standards value Western learning and technical know-how more than traditional sex differences. Those women who do achieve advanced Western education are in a superior position vis-à-vis men in regard to getting jobs with commercial enterprise, government, etc.

This creates problems for men—for one thing they resist employment of women in superior positions, and themselves resent working under women. For another, some begin to value educated women as hostesses and romantic sex partners in town, while maintaining traditional wives and families in the country. Thus, men seek to satisfy their new leanings toward individualism and Western standards as regards desirable women—literate, sophisticated—and their family's conservative push for maintaining traditional ties with rural customs. As Little says, "In West African countries, one of the problems is the uncertainty of the literate woman's position once she has moved out of the traditional family system." What are these women to do as they grow older, but without the extended kinship ties to insure their well-being?

When the African independence movements were at their height in the 1950s and 1960s, women got the vote, and there was a general euphoria about women's rights. Now the honeymoon period is over, and women are finding their independence more illusory than real. Cultural attitudes in places like Kenya, according to Little, are that women are not believed capable of political office. They are considered "big headed, power hungry, naïve, potentially unstable, weak charactered, and opportunistic," as if men were any different. Still women are running fashionable shops, small businesses, hold junior executive positions, and are university graduates in increasing numbers—how their lives will be affected by the mid-years is difficult to predict. This is the first generation to strike out beyond traditional family systems, where single women work in careers beyond those of traditional life, without the role models or traditions of male friends rather than lovers.

Such women are likely to fall back on the old system to keep them as they age. Women who have gone to live in the towns and become wealthy there, often return to their rural origins. But, since they had left, they do not have the children like other women their age who remained in traditional life styles. These returning women convert their capital into cattle, and adopt boys and girls of their own, in this way accumulating the family most people depend on in their later years for support and care. They give dowries to the girls and enrich the boys. They also distribute wealth to their paternal and maternal kin.

Other women, as well, are not ready to give up old family forms. For example, in a study of rural-urban residence and modernism in Ankara Province, Turkey, 1,138 married women in Ankara City and four rural villages were interviewed. It was found that the urban women were more modern, *but* the relative importance of extended family ties remained.[5]

Will the breakdown in traditional roles for older people in our society make us more happy or unhappy? What are the new life styles we can look forward to?

That inimitable comedienne, Sophie Tucker, used to say, "I've been rich and I've been poor, and rich is better." And it seems, contrary to what so many believe—money doesn't buy happiness—that money may indeed make one happier. Does age make a difference? She might have said, "I've been young and I've been old, and young is better"—or that traditional comment, "Youth is wasted on the young." Maybe youth is better for many things, especially the prospect of a long future stretching ahead, but in this case, youth, unlike money, makes very little difference concerning whether a person feels happy or sad.

Recent studies of mood as an indication of happiness, which looked at 6,552 persons aged four to ninety-nine, seemed to bear this out. The studies had interrupted people at leisure, home, and school and asked to assess their moods as happy, unhappy, or neutral. The researchers attempted to find the association between moods with age, sex, social class, and situational differences—what was happening to the people at the time they were asked to express their feelings. They found that, on the whole, women reported more moods of happiness and unhappiness than did men, compared with a neutral feeling. Interestingly, people, on the whole, reported being unhappy only 10 per cent of the time. Mood did not vary as a function of age! Middle-aged women were, therefore, found not to be any happier, unhappier, or neutral than women of other ages.[6]

The results, however, do bear out Sophie Tucker's experience. People of higher socioeconomic status reported more happiness—more money and higher position help. Significantly, people of all classes who were at *leisure* when interviewed reported more happiness than people at home, work, or school. This doesn't seem to support the notion that retirement and lack of "something to do" are necessarily the precursors of trouble and unhappiness. Our culture increasingly values leisure, and we appear to be less guilty about enjoying ourselves. It helps to have the money to do so.

Perhaps it is not necessary for women at mid-life and beyond to be particularly useful. Kenneth Galbraith, the economist, has suggested that our affluent society can support the nonproductive poor. Well, why not the nonproductive older adult? In our leisure-valuing society, to be able after years of toil to enjoy a period of play, mountains and seashore, golf and tennis, and no babies to watch may indeed be possible, and our leisure communities—no one under fifty allowed— seem to be headed in this direction for those who can afford them.

But there are others who deplore idleness and find absence of work demeaning and who resist isolation from the young. How to utilize the willing, able, and ready older people is a real challenge for our society, so wasteful of human energies. Certainly, to force retirement from work and society on the capable is to cause much waste and suffering.

Then there are those women who have devoted adult lifetimes to tasks they considered useful, but now devalued—housewife and mother—searching for the fulfillment of other social roles made impossible by their earlier acceptance of a particular definition of femininity. Are we ready to provide the tools and the facilities for further growth and development of these women? Will the welcome mat go out for older women in employment?

And there are the women who grew up with one set of values and morals, but now, in their maturity, are searching eagerly to pursue the newer or different styles of a changing world, and the new experiences to accompany them.

That our society is not ready with the answers to a good life for all is not surprising. The many different traditions that go into the makeup of modern populations carry with them different attitudes and values concerning aging; modern life conditions impose great changes upon those traditions. And the fact remains that there never before has been the need to confront the situation of such vast numbers of people living into and beyond middle age.

Menopause does not mean moving into old age—a whole new social era stretches out before we become really physically old. What to do with this period of life is something this generation of women must consider, for their experience will set the stage for their daughters who follow. The old negative patterns are not useful—but the lessons of those societies that teach the value of sex as play, the value of maturity as temperate wisdom, and provide useful roles for women have taught that there is nothing inevitable about demise with aging. "The best years of our lives" are, in reality, those we are experiencing. They are the only time we can be sure we have. To grasp the opportunity for enriched contact with life through friendships, activities, and new social roles is in order.

Choice and the expansion of choice regarding life style is typical of modern times. Limitations are placed by the values, resiliency, and experiences we bring with us to this period of our lives, as well as the economic ability to act in ways we desire. The world out there is not always ready to accept us on our terms. But the openness of choice nonetheless remains greater than ever before in the history of mankind. Errors, disappointments, carelessness can be expected as we grope for ways to live fully for the future. The "second season" has many pluses—having survived, in the first place, and having experienced growth and maturity, knowing that life is precious and should be treasured, and that people need to be kind to each other. Now other roles and different experiences can be explored, extending life into new dimensions. The negatives are not exclusively the province of women. Women and men together face the reality of their mortality, economic insecurity, and social values that have glorified youth and demeaned age. Women and men of all ages together will have to resist those values and those conditions as they assert their vitality.

We are thrust into dependence upon ourselves to carve out the possibility of graceful movement through all phases of the life cycle for ourselves and for those to follow in this new world of prolonged life for so many. Tolerance and pleasure in the many different life styles from which to choose is the way. So—ENJOY!

# CHAPTER REFERENCE NOTES

## Chapter I. Middle Age—Where It's At

1. Demographic data for this and the following chapters are drawn from various sources including: U. S. Department of Commerce, Bureau of the Census, *United States Census 1970, and Current Population Reports;* U. S. Department of Health, Education, and Welfare, National Center for Health Statistics; U. S. Department of Labor, Employment Standards Administration Women's Bureau; and Committee on Work and Personality in the Middle Years, Social Science Research Council.

Ethnographic data are drawn from the Human Area Relations File, personal field experiences, and specific literature referred to in the following chapters.

## Chapter II. Women and Sex—Here to Stay

1. Mark Twain, *Letters from the Earth*, ed: Bernard DeVoto (New York: Harper & Row, 1962), p. 40.

2. Ibid., p. 41.

3. Albert C. Kinsey, et al., *Sexual Behavior in the Human Female* (Philadelphia: W. B. Saunders Co., 1953), p. 353.

4. *Journal of Linnaeus*, quoted in Wilfrid Blunt, *The Compleat Naturalist* (New York: The Viking Press, 1971).

5. E. Jensen Krige and J. D. Krige, *The Realm of a Rain-Queen*, A Study of the Pattern of Lovedu Society (London: Oxford University Press, 1943), p. 158.

6. My own first anthropological field work was in this area and helped shape my perceptions of male-female relationships in our own society.

7. John S. Haller, Jr., "From Maidenhood to Menopause: Sex Education for Women in Victorian America," *Journal of Popular Culture*, pp. 49–70.

8. Quoted in Ibid.

9. Sula Benet, *How to Live to Be 100* (New York: Dial Press, 1976).

10. Erik Pfeiffer, M.D., "Sex and Aging," *Sexual Behavior* 2, No. 10 (October 1972), pp. 17–21.

11. William H. Masters, M.D., and Virginia E. Johnson, *Human Sexual Response* (New York: Little Brown, 1966).

12. William H. Masters, M.D., and Virginia E. Johnson, *Human Sexual Inadequacy* (New York: Little Brown, 1970), p. 342.

13. Diana Scully and Pauline Bart, "A Funny Thing Happened on the Way to the Orifice: Women in Gynecology Textbooks," in *Changing Women in a Changing Society*, ed: John Huber (Chicago: University of Chicago Press, 1973), pp. 283–87.

14. David Reuben, M.D., *Everything You Always Wanted to Know about Sex but Were Afraid to Ask* (New York: David McKay, 1969), p. 41.

15. Claude Lévi-Strauss, *The Raw and the Cooked* (New York: Harper & Row, 1975).

16. Sherry B. Ortner, "Is Female to Male as Nature is to Culture?" in *Women, Culture, and Society,* ed: M. Z. Rosaldo and L. Lamphere (Stanford, Calif.: Stanford University Press, 1974).

## Chapter III. Men and the Middle Years

1. *United States Census,* 1970.

2. Ruth Benedict, "Discontinuities in Cultural Conditioning," *Psychiatry,* May 1939, pp. 161–67.

3. Gerald B. Phillips, M.D., "Relationship Between Serum Sex Hormones and Glucose, Insulin, and Lipid Abnormalities in Men with Myocardial Infarction," *Proceedings of the National Academy of Sciences, U.S.A.,* Vol. 74 No. 4 (April 1972), pp. 1729–33.

4. D. A. Hamburg and B. Hamburg, "Occupational Stress, Endocrine Changes, and Coping Behavior in the Middle Years of Adult Life," unpublished paper prepared for the Committee on Work and Personality in the Middle Years, Social Science Research Council.

5. Sula Benet, *How to Live to Be 100* (New York: Dial Press, 1976).

6. Bernice Neugarten, *Middle Age and Aging: A Reader in Social Psychology* (Chicago: University of Chicago Press, 1968).

7. *Newsweek,* July 4, 1976.

8. Ibid.

9. Martha Weinman Lear, "Is There a Male Menopause?" New York *Times Magazine,* January 28, 1973.

10. Orville G. Brim, Jr., "Theories of the Male Mid-Life Crisis," *The Counseling Psychologist,* 6, No. 1 (1976), pp. 2–9.

11. Ibid., p. 5.

12. Morton Kramer and Richard W. Redich, "Epidemiological Indices in the Middle Years," paper prepared for the Committee on Work and Personality in the Middle Years, Social Science Research Council, 1974.

13. Brim, op. cit., p. 5.

14. Ibid.

15. D. Gutman, "The Country of Old Men—Cross-Cultural Studies in the Psychology of Later Life," in *Occasional Papers in Gerontology,* ed: W. Donahue (Ann Arbor: University of Michigan, 1969).

16. Kramer and Redich, op. cit.

17. Bernice Neugarten and N. Datan, "Sociological Perspectives on the Life Cycle," in *Life Span Developmental Psychology: Personality and Socialization,* ed: P. B. Baltes and K. W. Schare (New York: Academic Press, 1973), pp. 53–69.

18. Joseph Heller, *Something Happened* (New York: Alfred Knopf, 1974).

19. Margaret Mead, quoted in Martha Weinman Lear, "Is There a Male Menopause?" New York *Times Magazine*, January 28, 1973.
20. Ibid.

## Chapter IV. The Beauty Industry—Friend or Enemy?

1. Doris Lessing, *Summer Before the Dark* (New York: Alfred Knopf, 1973).
2. Jane Richardson and A. L. Kroeber, "Three Centuries of Women's Dress," *Anthropological Record*, 1940; Edward Sapir, "Fashion," *Encyclopedia of the Social Sciences*, Vol. 6 (New York: Macmillan Co., 1931), pp. 139–44.
3. "100 Years of Good Looks," *McCall's* magazine, April 1976, p. 22.
4. Mary Wollstonecraft, A *Vindication of the Rights of Women* (England: Penguin Books, 1974; originally written in 1792).
5. Murray Wax, "Themes in Cosmetics and Grooming," *The American Journal of Sociology*, 62, No. 6 (May 1957), pp. 558–93.
6. Maria Kresz, "The Community of Young People in a Transylvanian Village," in *Youth in a Changing World*, ed: Estelle Fuchs (The Hague: Mouton Publishers, 1976), pp. 207–12.
7. George Simmel, "The Sociology of Sociability," trans. from the German by Everett C. Hughes, *American Journal of Sociology* (November 1940), pp. 254–61.

## Chapter V. A Social "Change of Life"

1. Arnold Van Gennep, *Rites de Passage* (Chicago: University of Chicago Press, 1960).
2. Doris Lessing, *Summer Before the Dark* (New York: Alfred Knopf, 1973).
3. Vieda Skulans, "Symbolic Significance of Menstruation and the Menopause," *Man*, New Series, 15 No. 4 (December 1970), pp. 639–51.
4. A point of view expressed by Helene Deutsch, M.D., *The Psychology of Women* (New York: Grune and Stratton, Vol. I, 1944; Vol. II, 1945); Lydia Sicher, M.D., Ph.D., "Change of Life, a Psychosomatic Problem," *American Journal of Psychotherapy* (September 1949), pp. 399–409.
5. Robert Murphy, "Social Distance and the Veil," *American Anthropologist* 66, No. 6 (December 1964), pp. 1257–74.
6. Pauline B. Bart, "Why Women's Status Changes in Middle Age," *Sociological Symposium*, No. 3 (Fall 1969).

## Chapter VI. The Many Roles of Women

1. U. S. Department of Labor, Employment Standard Administration, Women's Bureau, *The Earnings Gap Between Women and Men*, 1976; U. S. Department of Labor, *Handbook on Women Workers*, Bulletin #297; U. S. Department of Labor, *Women in 1975*; U. S. Department of Commerce, Bureau of the Census, Current Population Reports Special Studies, A *Statistical Portrait of*

*Women in the U.S.*, Special Studies Series P23, No. 58 (Washington, D.C.: U. S. Government Printing Office, 1976).

2. Center for the American Woman and Politics, Eagleton Institute of Politics, Rutgers University, *Women in Public Affairs* (Ann Arbor, Mich.: R. R. Bowker, 1976).

3. M. Z. Rosaldo, "A Theoretical Overview," in *Women, Culture, and Society*, ed: M. Z. Rosaldo and L. Lamphere (Stanford, Calif.: Stanford University Press, 1974), p. 29.

4. Joel Aronoff and Wm. D. Crano, "A Re-examination of the Cross-Cultural Principles of Task Segregation and Sex Role Differentiation in the Family," *American Sociological Review* 40 (February 1975), pp. 12–20.

5. E. Campbell, *Honor, Family, and Patronage* (London: Oxford University Press, 1964).

6. Monique Gessain, "Coniagu Women," in *Women of Tropical Africa*, ed: Denise Paulme, trans. H. M. Wright (Berkeley and Los Angeles: University of California Press, 1971), p. 11.

7. David C. Gordon, "Women of Algeria, an Essay on Change," *Harvard Middle Eastern Monographs*, 19 (Cambridge, Mass.: Center for Middle Eastern Studies, 1968).

8. M. Zborowski and E. G. Herzog, *Life is with People* (New York: International University Press, 1952).

9. Radcliffe-Brown, *Structure and Function in Primitive Society* (New York: Free Press, 1952), p. 103.

10. Michael Young and Peter Willmott, *Family and Kinship in East London* (London: Routledge and Kegan Paul, 1957).

11. Frances L. K. Hsu, *Under the Ancestor's Shadow* (New York: Columbia University Press, 1948), p. 59.

12. Henny Harald Hansen, *Daughters of Allah, Among Moslem Women in Kurdistan* (London: Ruskin House, George Allen and Unwin, Ltd., 1960).

13. Vitold de Golish, *Primitive India* (London: George G. Harrap and Co., 1954), p. 18.

14. Pauline B. Bart, "Why Women's Status Changes in Middle Age," *Sociological Symposium*, No. 3, Fall 1969.

15. New York *Times*, June 11, 1976.

16. Marabel Morgan, *The Total Woman* (New York: Pocket Books, 1975).

17. Morris, 1854, quoted in Ann F. Scott, *The Southern Lady from Pedestal to Politics 1830–1930* (Chicago: University of Chicago Press, 1970).

18. Ann Oakley, *The Sociology of Housework* (New York: Pantheon Books, 1974); Ann Oakley, *The Housewife, Past and Present* (New York: Pantheon Books, 1974).

19. Alan C. Kerkoff, "Family Patterns and Morale in Retirement," in *Social Aspects of Aging*, ed: Ida H. Simpson and John C. McKinney (Durham, N.C.: Duke University Press, 1966).

20. New York *Times*, June 12, 1976.

21. E. Jensen Krige and J. D. Krige, *The Realm of a Rain-Queen*, A Study of the Pattern of Lovedu Society (London: Oxford University Press, 1943).

22. Carol Hoffer, "Acquisition and Exercise of Political Power by a Woman

Paramount Chief of the Sherbro People" (Ph.D. dissertation, Bryn Mawr College, 1971); "Mende and Sherbro Women in High Office," *Canadian Journal of African Studies* 6, No. 2 (1972), pp. 151–64.

## Chapter VII. Menopause—When

1. Jane C. Goodale, *Tiwi Wives* (Seattle and London: University of Washington Press, 1971).

2. D. W. Amundsen and C. J. Diers, "The Age of Menopause in Classical Greece and Rome," *Human Biology*, 42, No. 79 (1970).

3. J. B. Post, "Ages at Menarche and Menopause: Some Mediaeval Authorities," *Population Studies* 25, No. 83 (1971), pp. 83–87; D. W. Amundsen and C. J. Diers, "The Age of Menopause in Medieval Europe, *Human Biology*, 45, No. 4 (1973), pp. 605–12.

4. G. Friere, "Mean Age at Menopause and Menarche in South Africa," *South African Journal of Medical Science* 36, No. 21 (1971).

5. J. M. Tanner, *Growth at Adolescence* (Oxford: Blackwell Scientific Publications, 1962).

6. Lawrence A. Malcolm, "Growth and Developmental Patterns and Human Differentiation in Papua New Guinean Communities," in *Youth in a Changing World*, ed: Estelle Fuchs (The Hague: Mouton Publishers, 1976).

7. Alan E. Treloar, "Menarche, Menopause and Intervening Fecundity," *Human Biology* 46, No. 1 (February 1974), pp. 89–107.

8. Marsha Flint, "Menarche and Menopause of Rajput Women" (Ph.D. dissertation, City University of New York, 1974).

9. A. Fusancha and P. Baker, "Attitude and Growth: a Study of the Patterns of Growth of a High Altitude Peruvian Quechua Population," *American Journal of Physical Anthropology* 32, No. 2 (March 1970), pp. 279–92.

10. Brian MacMahon and J. Worcester, *Ages at Menopause, 1960–1962*, National Center for Health Statistics, U. S. Department of Health, Education and Welfare, Public Health Service Series 11, No. 19 (Washington, D.C.: U. S. Government Printing Office, 1966).

11. M. Kamal and R. Kamal, "Diet and Fecundity in India," paper presented at the Sixth International Conference on Planned Parenthood, New Delhi, February, 1959.

12. MacMahon and Worcester, op. cit.

13. A. F. Currier, *The Menopause* (New York: Appleton, 1897).

14. E. Heinrich Kisch, *The Sexual Life of Women and the Physiological and Hygienic Aspects*, trans. from German by M. Paul (New York: Allied Book Co., 1928).

15. Marie Carmichael Stopes, *Change of Life in Men and Women* (London: Putnam Publications, 1936).

16. Carl Wood, "The Female Reproductive System," in *The Health of a Metropolis, the Findings of the Melbourne Metropolitan Health and Social Survey*, ed: Jerzy Krupinski and Allan Stoller (Sydney, Australia: Halsted Press, 1971), pp. 52–60.

17. G. A. Hauser, et al., "Menarche and Menopause in Israel," *Gynaecologia* 155, No. 39 (1963).

## *Chapter* VIII. Menopause—A "Biological Change of Life"—The Physiological Facts

1. The physiology of the menopause is discussed in: Edmund R. Novak, M.D., et al., *Textbook of Gynecology*, 8th ed. (Baltimore: Williams & Wilkins Co., 1970); R. W. Kistner, *Principles and Practices of Gynecology*, 2nd ed. (Chicago: Year Book Medical Publishers, 1971); Boston Women's Health Book Collective, *Our Bodies Ourselves* (New York: Simon and Schuster, 1971).

2. William E. Easterling, Jr., M.D., "Managing the Menopause," *American Family Physician* 7, No. 3 (March 1973), p. 139.

3. Rena Gropper and Sula Benet, personal communication.

4. Vieda Skulans, "Symbolic Significance of Menstruation and the Menopause," *Man*, New Series, 15 No. 4 (December 1970), pp. 639–51.

5. Doris T. Williams, personal communication.

## *Chapter* IX. Menopause—Is It Necessary? The Search for Immortality and the Estrogen Controversy

1. Edmund R. Novak, M.D., et al., *Textbook of Gynecology*, 8th ed. (Baltimore: Williams & Wilkins Co., 1970), p. 626.

2. R. A. Wilson, M.D., *Feminine Forever* (New York: Pocket Books, 1968); R. A. Wilson, "Specific Procedures for the Elimination of the Menopause," *Western Journal of Surgery* 71 (1968), p. 100.

3. David Reuben, M.D., *Everything You Always Wanted to Know about Sex but Were Afraid to Ask* (New York: David McKay, 1969). Dr. Reuben reversed himself on this point in later works.

4. Ibid., p. 41.

5. M. Dorothea Kerr, M.D., "Psychohormonal Approach to the Menopause," *Modern Treatment* 5, No. 3 (May 1968), pp. 587–95; "Psychohormonal Treatment During the Menopause," *American Family Physician* (February 1975); *Vogue* (January 1974). In *Vogue*, Dr. Kerr glibly wrote, ". . . cancer is a needless fear in women taking estrogen," p. 103.

6. M. Dorothea Kerr, M.D., "Emotional/Hormonal Aspects of the Menopause," *The Female Climacteric* (n.p. Ayerst Laboratories, 1972).

7. Noel S. Weiss, M.D., et al., "Increasing Incidence of Endometrial Cancer in the United States," *The New England Journal of Medicine* 294, No. 23 (June 1976), pp. 1259–62.

8. Boston Collaborative Drug Surveillance Program, "Estrogen and Gall Bladder Diseases, Venous Thromboembolism, and Breast Tumors in Relation to Postmenopausal Estrogen Therapy," *The New England Journal of Medicine* 290, No. 1 (January 1974), pp. 51–52.

9. Thomas M. Mack, M.D., "Estrogens and Endometrial Cancer in a Retire-

ment Community," *The New England Journal of Medicine* 294, No. 23 (June 1976), pp. 1262–67.

10. *New York Times*, January 20, 1976.

11. K. J. Lennane and R. J. Lennane, "Alleged Psychogenic Disorders in Women, a Possible Manifestation of Sexual Prejudice," *New England Journal of Medicine* 288 (1973), p. 288.

12. Sonja M. McKinlay and John B. McKinlay, "Selected Studies of the Menopause," *Journal of Biosocial Science* 5 (1973), p. 534.

13. Ibid., p. 535.

14. J. R. Clayden, et al., "Menopause Flushing—Double Blind Trial of a Non-Hormonal Medication," *British Medical Journal* 1 (March 1974), pp. 409–12.

15. G. Rybo and H. Westerberg, "Symptoms in the Postmenopause—a Population Study," *Acta Obstetrica et Gynecologica Scandinavica* 50 (1971), p. 25.

16. Ibid.

17. Martin J. Kelly, Jr., "Who Me—a Sexist?" *New England Journal of Medicine* 288, No. 6 (1973), pp. 317–18.

18. Lennane and Lennane, op. cit.

19. Robert Bergman, "Medication Abuse by Middle-Aged Women," *Social Casework* 54 (1975), pp. 526–32.

20. *New York Times*, May 27, 1976.

## Chapter x. Pregnancy and Babies

1. Rena Gropper, *Gypsies in the City* (Princeton, N.J.: Darwin Press, 1975).

2. Sula Benet, *How to Live to Be 100* (New York: Dial Press, 1976).

3. *New York Times*, August 27, 1976.

4. *New York Times*, December 6, 1976.

## Chapter xi. You Don't Go Crazy at Menopause

1. Margaret Mead, *Coming of Age in Samoa* (New York: William Morrow, 1928).

2. Estelle Fuchs, ed., *Youth in a Changing World* (The Hague: Mouton Publishers, 1976).

3. M. Dorothea Kerr, "Psychohormonal Approach to the Menopause," *Modern Treatment* 5, No. 3 (May 1968).

4. George Winokur, "Depression in the Menopause," *American Journal of Psychiatry* 130 (January 1973), pp. 92–93.

5. Jacqueline Susann, *Once Is Not Enough* (New York: Bantam Books, 1973), p. 296.

6. Gilbert Cant, "Valiumania," *New York Times Magazine*, February 1, 1976.

7. Michelle Zimbalist Rosaldo, "A Theoretical Overview," in *Women, Culture, and Society,* ed: Michelle Zimbalist Rosaldo and Louise Lamphere (Stanford, Calif.: Stanford University Press, 1974).

8. K. Stern and M. Prados, "Personality Studies in Menopausal Women," *American Journal of Psychiatry* 103 (1946), p. 358.

9. Ibid.

10. Helene Deutsch, "The Psychiatric Component in Gynaecology," in *Neuroses and Character Types* (London: Hogarth Press, 1965).

11. Vieda Skulans, "The Symbolic Significance of Menstruation and the Menopause," *Man*, New Series, 15 No. 4 (December 1970), pp. 639–51.

12. Helene Deutsch, *The Psychology of Women* (New York: Grune and Stratton, Vol. I, 1944, Vol. II, 1945).

13. Lydia Sicher, M.D., Ph.D., "Change of Life, a Psychosomatic Problem," *American Journal of Psychotherapy* (September 1949), pp. 399–409.

14. Ernest Becker, "Social Science and Psychiatry," *Antioch Review* 23 (1963), pp. 353–65.

## Chapter XII. Middle Age and Health—Women Are Mortal

1. Current Population Reports, Special Studies, U. S. Department of Commerce, Bureau of the Census, *A Statistical Portrait of Women in the U.S.*, Special Studies Series P23, No. 58 (Washington, D.C.: U. S. Government Printing Office, 1976).

2. Current Population Reports, U. S. Department of Commerce, Bureau of the Census, *Demographic Aspects of Aging and the Older Population in the United States*, Special Studies Series P23, No. 59 (Washington, D.C.: U. S. Government Printing Office, n.d.).

3. Ibid., and Ashley Montague, *The Natural Superiority of Women*, new rev. ed. (New York: Collier Books, 1974).

4. Robert H. Furman, M.D. "Coronary Heart Disease in the Menopause," in *Menopause and Aging*, ed: K. J. Ryan and D. C. Gibson, MPH, U. S. Department of Health, Education and Welfare, National Institute of Health, National Institute of Child Development and Human Development (Washington, D.C.: U. S. Government Printing Office, n.d.), pp. 73–319.

5. Gordon Hems, "The Menopause and Breast Cancer," *The Lancet* 1 (1974), p. 362.

6. Ibid.

7. New York *Times*, January 21, 1976.

8. New York *Times*, December 6, 1976.

9. Robert W. Cali, M.D., "Management of the Climacteric and Postmenopausal Woman," *Symposium on Therapeutic Problems* 58, No. 3 (May 1972), pp. 789–99.

10. Edmund R. Novak, et al., *Textbook of Gynecology*, 8th ed. (Baltimore: Williams & Wilkins Co., 1970).

11. *The Medical Letter on Drugs and Therapeutics* 15, No. 2 (issue 366) (January 1973). (New Rochelle, N.Y.: The Medical Letter, Inc.)

## Chapter XIII. Hysterectomy—The Chances Are
## You Won't Need One

1. Rates based on estimates from the "Hospital Discharge Survey (1974)," Division of Health Resources Utilization Statistics, U. S. Department of Health, Education, and Welfare.

2. Jack Batten, "Is This Operation Necessary?" *Chatelaine* 48, No. 8 (August 1975), pp. 48–59.

3. Commission on Professional and Hospital Activities.

4. James C. Doyle, "Unnecessary Hysterectomies," *Journal of the American Medical Association* 151 (1952), pp. 360–65.

5. Ray S. Trussell and Mildred Moorehead, *The Quantity, Quality, and Costs of Medical and Hospital Care Secured by a Sample of Teamster Families in the New York Area* (New York: Columbia University School of Public Health and Administrative Medicine, 1962).

6. Eugene G. McCarthy, M.D., M.P.H. and Ann Susan Kamons, "Mandatory and Voluntary Second Opinion Programs in the Greater New York area with National Implications," The Dorothy R. Eisenberg Lecture, Department of Surgery, Harvard Medical School, June 12, 1976.

7. Batten, op. cit.

8. Alfred C. Kinsey, et al., *Sexual Behavior in the Human Female* (Philadelphia: W. B. Saunders Co., 1953), p. 735.

9. Quoted in Batten, op. cit., p. 48.

10. Ibid., pp. 57–58.

11. Dr. Walter Alvarez, personal communication.

12. Vieda Skulans, "Symbolic Significance of Menstruation and the Menopause," *Man*, New Series 15, No. 4 (December 1970), pp. 639–51.

13. Barbara Goldstein of NOW, quoted in Joanne Rodgers, "The Rush to Surgery," New York *Times Magazine*, September 21, 1975.

14. Dr. Herbert S. Denenberg, *A Shopper's Guide to Surgery* (Valley Forge, Pa.: National Liberty Corporation, 1975).

15. Quoted in Ibid.

16. *Accreditation Manual for Doctors* (Chicago: Joint Commission on Accreditation of Hospitals, 1976).

17. George J. Ames, *Rights of Hospital Patients* (New York: Avon Books, 1974).

## *Chapter* XIV. Divorce and Widowhood—on Being Alone

1. Jessie Bernard, "Introduction," in *Divorce and After*, ed: Paul Bohannan (Garden City: Doubleday-Anchor, 1971).

2. *McCall's* magazine, April 1976.

3. New York *Times*, May 24, 1976.

4. Jessie Bernard, "Infidelity, a Moral or Social Issue," *Science and Psychoanalysis*, 16 (1970), pp. 99–126.

5. Paul Bohannan, "The Six Stations of Divorce," in *Divorce and After*, ed: Bohannan, pp. 33–62.

6. Morton M. Hunt, *The World of the Formerly Married* (New York: McGraw-Hill, 1966).

7. Henny Harald Hansen, *Daughters of Allah, Among Moslem Women in Kurdistan* (London: Ruskin House, George Allen and Unwin, Ltd., 1960).

8. Paul Gebhard, "Postmarital Coitus Among Widows and Divorcees," in *Divorce and After*, ed: Bohannan, p. 98.

9. Shere Hite, *The Hite Report* (New York: Macmillan, 1976).

10. Ernest S. Burch, Jr., "Marriage Among the North Alaskan Eskimo," in *Divorce and After*, ed: Bohannan, pp. 171–204.

11. Ronald Cohen, *The Kanuri of Bornu* (New York: Holt, Rinehart, & Winston, 1967).

12. Paul C. Rosenblatt, et al., *Grief and Mourning in Cross-cultural Perspective* (New Haven: Human Relations Area File Press, 1976).

## *Chapter* xv. Growing Older Is in Style

1. Quoted in New York *Times*, June 1, 1976.

2. Alex Inkeles and David H. Smith, *Becoming Modern, Individual Change in Six Developing Countries* (Cambridge: Harvard University Press, 1974).

3. Estelle Fuchs, ed., *Youth in a Changing World* (The Hague: Mouton Publishers, 1976).

4. Kenneth Little, *African Women in Towns* (Cambridge: Cambridge University Press, 1973).

5. Allen Schnaiberg, "Rural-Urban Residence and Modernism," *Demography*, 7 (February 1970), pp. 71–85.

6. Paul Cameron, "Mood as an Indicant of Happiness: Age, Sex, Social Class, and Situational Differences," *Journal of Gerontology* 30 (March 1975), pp. 216–24.

# Appendix

## A SHOPPER'S GUIDE TO SURGERY*

### *Fourteen Rules On How To Avoid Unnecessary Surgery*

#### PREFACE

Too many people (some say up to two million a year or more in the United States) are subjecting themselves to unnecessary surgery. They often do so without adequate investigation or consideration.

Dr. Paul R. Hawley, a famous medical authority and surgeon, has said: "I shall never cease to be astonished at the number of people who would not invest a penny in any enterprise without full assurance of its safety, yet who will hop on the operating table and permit anyone to cut into their bellies."

Unnecessary surgery takes a needless toll of human lives and generates suffering, disability and expense.

Many studies have documented our national scandal of unnecessary surgery. One of the most noteworthy of these studies was conducted in 1962 to 1964 by the Columbia University School of Public Health and Administrative Medicine. The group surveyed various types of surgery. It found, for example, that of 60 hysterectomies, "⅓ of the patients were operated on unnecessarily and that question could be raised on the advisability of the operation in another 10 percent." Of 13 caesarean sections (delivery of a baby by means of an abdominal operation), there were serious questions about the necessity of surgery in 7 cases. There is every reason to believe that the conclusions of the Columbia study are still valid.

A Ralph Nader group in 1971 as well as other independent investigations have reached the same conclusion. Dr. Charles E. Lewis, a Harvard specialist in community health, concluded a 1969 study of the incidence of surgery with this comment: "The results presented might be interpreted as supporting a medical variation of Parkinson's law: patient

* Reproduced with permission of the Pennsylvania Insurance Department

admissions for surgery expand to fill beds, operating suites and surgeon's time." And there is an abundance of professional opinion that unnecessary surgery is widespread. Dr. John Knowles, now President of the Rockefeller Foundation, in 1972, warned that "incredible amounts of unnecessary surgery are going on" (Baltimore *Sun*, May 29, 1972, page 4).

This short "Shopper's Guide to Surgery" is intended to give the public some basic rules on how to avoid unnecessary surgery. It is also intended to give the consumer the kind of information he needs to help hold down the cost of health care and to better utilize the health delivery system.

This Guide was originally published as part of the "Shopper's Guide" Series of the Pennsylvania Insurance Department.

Ralph Nader, the leading consumer advocate, has called on other Insurance Commissioners to follow our lead and prepare Guides of their own. We think that's an excellent suggestion. We also think it would be sound for consumer and industry groups to start following suit. It's about time the consumer gets the facts. It's about time we make our free enterprise system of competition work like it's supposed to. It's about time we give the public the facts. We think these "Shopper's Guides" are a step in the right direction.

We know that an informed public will be in a better position to make decisions regarding its own health and welfare. We believe that one of the tasks of government is to inform the public. An informed public will help to prevent abuses that now plague the consumer. These informational "Guides," therefore, have an important place in the regulatory processes of government.

This "Guide" follows the original June 1972 publication except for minor editorial changes necessary to shift from a Pennsylvania to a national focus.

As future editions of this "Guide" are contemplated, we would greatly appreciate receiving suggestions for improving it. Send them to Herbert S. Denenberg, P.O. Box 146, Wynnewood, Pennsylvania 19096.

Herbert S. Denenberg, Ph.D.
*Former Pennsylvania Insurance Commissioner*
*July, 1975*

## A SHOPPER'S GUIDE TO SURGERY

Some authorities estimate there are as many as 2,000,000 unnecessary surgical operations in the United States each year. How to decide if the surgery you've been asked to undergo fits the category of the 2,000,000 unnecessary operations or the 10,000,000 necessary ones is the purpose of this "Guide."

Don't assume you can place blind trust in our system of medical care. Ralph Nader has pointed out: "Conditions of medical care are often criminally negligent especially for the poor and even at times for the relatively affluent. The endless reports of such conditions by physicians, government investigations and other reliable inquiries and testimony present macabre scenes so repeatedly that they invoke resigned or indifferent responses. The rocketing cost of health care with the advent of socialized payment of physicians' bills through Medicare has not improved the quality of care, but it has enriched the medical profession to an unprecedented degree."

You are placing undue trust in our medical care system if you assume one doctor is as good as another, or that any doctor can provide you with the quality medical care you need. Many doctors, some 15,000 nationally, are licensed but unfit to practice medicine according to conservative estimates, as reported in a 1970 book by Howard R. and Martha E. Lewis called *The Medical Offenders*. Many doctors may be qualified to render medical care, but may be totally unqualified to perform surgery.

This "Guide" should help you find a qualified surgeon when you need one. It should also enable you to take other needed steps to avoid unnecessary surgery.

You can't diagnose your own case, but there are some simple rules you can apply to make sure that you really need the surgery that might be prescribed.

## Rule 1

Don't go directly to a surgeon for medical treatment. If at all possible, start out by going to a general practitioner or internist. Go to your regular family doctor—a general practitioner or internist—for any initial diagnosis or treatment. Unfortunately, there is a shortage of general practitioners and a surplus of surgeons.

You will also need a general practitioner or internist to treat you after the surgery and to work with your surgeon in providing care both before and after surgery. Everyone should have a family doctor, who is a general practitioner or internist, and you should get one before you're sick. Don't wait until you urgently need one. Select one so he'll be available the minute he's needed. Also, you want him to have time to know you and learn your medical history. Develop a good relationship with a family doctor. He will then be able to provide you with better care and he'll be more likely to save you from unnecessary surgery.

Most surgeons are competent, conscientious, careful and conservative, as are most other physicians. Some are narrowly trained and tend to do what they are trained to do—operate. A small minority are knife-happy, incompetent and greedy. And there is a tendency for surgeons to do their thing—which is to perform surgery.

Even in the case of a superb surgeon, a general practitioner or internist can often serve as a countervailing force on any tendency of a surgeon to place too much faith in surgery.

This tendency of medical men (such as general practitioners and internists) to be more conservative than surgeons is documented in Dr. William A. Nolen's best seller, *The Making of A Surgeon*:

*Kevin Jonas (a surgeon) was, naturally, eager to do some heart cases. He would gladly have paid a thousand dollars apiece for potential patients even if he'd have had to steal to get the money, but of course there weren't any for sale. He had to depend on the medical men and they weren't eager to have their patients operated upon. Internists don't take kindly to new surgical procedures; they're from Missouri when it comes to surgical pioneering—as, I suppose, they should be.*

Christiaan Barnard, the famed heart transplanter, in his autobiography, relates how eager he was to find a patient for a heart transplant. "Maybe we were too anxious," he writes. He catalogues his considerable discomfort while eagerly awaiting the first heart transplant operation:

*All through the last two weeks of October I kept after Professor Schrire—plaguing him day and night. The delay and subsequent anxiety caused an alarming flare-up in my arthritis. Both hands and feet began to swell and with such pain I feared it would prevent me from operating when Professor Schrire finally decided to release a patient.*

There is some tendency for too much surgery when there are too many surgeons around. It is no mere coincidence that in proportion to population, U.S. surgeons not only are twice as numerous as English surgeons, but also perform twice as many operations.

An authoritative study in 1970 by Dr. John P. Bunker concluded that there is a disproportionately large number of surgeons in the United States and this may lead to some unnecessary surgery. An editorial published in the June, 1972 issue of the *Archives of Surgery*, a publication of the American Medical Association, confirmed that we have a surplus of surgeons.

## Rule 2

Make sure any surgeon that is to perform surgery on you is Board certified. This means his competence as a surgeon has been certified by one of the American Specialty Boards, after a vigorous oral, written and clinical examination. There are about 51,000 surgeons who are Board certified.

One authority, Dr. Robert E. Rothenberg, a well-known surgeon, in his book *Understanding Surgery*, has concluded: "It is safe to say that an American Specialty Board diploma in a doctor's office is almost a guarantee of his efficiency." For some reason, Dr. Rothenberg said nothing of a guarantee of conscience or character. His statement may be too sweeping an endorsement, but a Board certified surgeon is still a sound minimum qualification. It is one important test of a surgeon's ability.

Osteopathic surgeons may be accredited by the American Specialty Board in some states or by their own American Osteopathic Board of Surgery.

There are competent surgeons who are not Board certified. If you want to use them, you should be careful to check them out all the more carefully by the other rules suggested here.

In some rural areas, Board certified surgeons may not be available. Under these circumstances, the patient may have to travel to a larger city if he cannot otherwise assure himself of the competency of those surgeons available locally.

You can find out for sure if a surgeon is Board certified by calling your local county medical society or using the Directory of Medical Specialists available in most good public libraries.

It pays to look for a competent surgeon. Some reliable experts, including Dr. Paul R. Hawley, have claimed that one half of the surgical operations in the U.S. are performed by surgeons who are inadequately trained to undertake such surgery. In June of 1972, Dr. Eric W. Fonkalsrud of the editorial board of the American Medical Association's *Archives of Surgery* said that about half of the operations in the country are being performed by doctors who are not Board certified surgeons.

One expert, Dr. Harold T. Hyman, in a widely used medical reference book, suggests that the patient not only check out the surgeon but also the anesthesiologist. Others would rely on the surgeon to see that a qualified anesthesiologist is selected for the surgery.

## Rule 3

Make sure the surgeon you are to use is a Fellow of the American College of Surgeons (F.A.C.S.). There are about 25,000 surgeons who are designated Fellows. The American College of Surgeons has membership qualifications that keep out the less competent surgeons, and the College also stresses programs of continuing education.

This is not an infallible rule, of course, but it is one that is well worth applying in selecting any surgeon.

You can check as to whether any surgeon is a Fellow of the American College of Surgeons in the same fashion as you check to see if he is Board-certified—consult the Directory of Medical Specialists or call your local county medical society. You can also write directly to the American College of Surgeons, 55 East Erie Street, Chicago, Illinois 60611.

The equivalent organization for Osteopaths is the American College of Osteopathic Surgeons located at 1550 South Dixie Highway, Suite 216, Coral Gables, Florida 33146.

## Rule 4

Even if your family doctor and surgeon agree that surgery is necessary, consider getting an independent consultation or opinion before subjecting yourself to surgery.

Consultations, according to some studies, reduce operations by as much as 20 to 60 percent. You may be in that 20 to 60 percent. And you have a right to seek consultation.

As one expert, writing under the pseudonym of Dr. Lawrence P. Williams, says in a book entitled *How to Avoid Unnecessary Surgery:*

*The old saying, two heads are better than one, is as true in medicine as anywhere else—possibly even more so, for conscientious doctors have found out that in order to present a problem case to another doctor, they must first review and organize the facts of the case. This in itself often makes the problem clearer. A second independent surgeon, moreover, may consider certain aspects of the condition quite differently, throwing a new light on the problem. The chance that other factors pertaining to the surgery will be brought out is greater with a consultation.*

The second doctor must be truly independent. He should not be part of a "you-scratch-my-back-I'll-scratch-your-back" arrangement. The second surgeon should be told his opinion is being sought but he will *not* do the surgery if it is necessary. This removes any financial incentive for him to suggest surgery.

for general anesthesia is a good example. If general anesthesia, which involves loss of consciousness, must be used, there is always significant risk. Death and complications from anesthesia are among the most serious risks arising from surgery. Any time general anesthesia is to be used, even an operation that merely involves a surface procedure without cutting into a body cavity, there is a significant risk.

As general anesthesia involves significant risk, it is preferable to have it administered by a physician anesthesiologist who is a specialist, or under his supervision by a certified, trained nurse anesthetist. It is a good idea to be sure the hospital you go to uses a physician anesthesiologist.

Perhaps the best definition of major surgery that puts the risk involved in true perspective is the one that goes like this: If it involves you, it may be minor surgery. If it involves me, it's major surgery.

You should also know what the alternatives to surgery are, such as diet in the case of a peptic ulcer. Surgery is typically a last resort, and you should be as sure as you can that you've explored all treatment short of surgery. Needless to say, you should know the benefits of the proposed surgery. You can hardly judge the risk or even the need for surgery without a clear picture of its likely benefits. Of course, if it is clear that surgery is needed, it should not be delayed to the point where further harm may result.

### Rule 8

Frankly discuss the fee for surgery with your doctor. You should know what the surgery is going to cost. Furthermore, most surgeons prefer that the patient understand the cost of surgery in advance. So, forget all about the mistaken notion that it's somewhat improper to inquire about cost of surgery.

Any surgeon worth his scalpel will gladly discuss fees. If he is not willing to do so, then he doesn't know much about his obligation to the patient and the patient's right to know.

Be sure you know all costs involved—the surgeon's fees, any fees for his assistant, the anesthesiologist's fees, those of the hospital, special nursing, your own physician's fees, and any other costs.

This discussion of fees will have several important incidental advantages.

It gives you a better idea of the nature of the surgery.

It also may suggest improper arrangements between the surgeon and assistant. If the assistant's fee is much beyond 20 percent of the surgeon's fee, it may suggest fee-splitting. For example, if the assistant is also a doctor, a high assistant's fee may suggest "fee-splitting," a form of medical kickback to the doctor from the surgeon. Don't put yourself

You may want to select the second surgeon on your own, or perhaps get recommendations from your family doctor or surgeon.

When a consultation is to be rendered, the first surgeon ordinarily briefs the second one on the case and his tentative diagnosis and recommendation.

Some would prefer a totally independent opinion rather than an independent consultation with the second surgeon working on his own and being unaware of the conclusions of the other surgeon. This may remove any tendency to be too quick about going down the wrong path with the first surgeon.

One well-known surgeon suggested that the best way to avoid unnecessary surgery is to get three independent opinions without advising any of the three surgeons involved about the conclusions of the other two.

How many consultations and opinions you should have depends on the facts and circumstances of each case. The need for additional consultations and opinions is a matter which you can discuss with your own doctor and surgeon. In some clear-cut cases (pardon this figure of speech), no consultation will be necessary at all. And of course, there may be need for emergency surgery—as, for example, after an auto accident or in the event of a ruptured appendix—when there may not be sufficient time to follow the rules suggested here.

If a doctor refuses to seek consultation upon request, he is violating the ethical rules of the medical profession. For example, Section 8 of the American Medical Association Principles of Medical Ethics states:

*A physician should seek consultation upon request; in doubtful or difficult cases; or whenever it appears that the quality of medical care may be enhanced thereby.*

Look out for a doctor or surgeon who is afraid of consultation or becomes angry or disturbed at the prospect of consultation. Drop a doctor or surgeon who can't accept another expert's consultation graciously. As between your doctor's or surgeon's ego and your health, opt for the latter.

If a doctor improperly refuses consultation, you can report his refusal to the county medical society for possible disciplinary action, as well as to appropriate state medical licensing authorities and consumer-protection agencies.

### Rule 5

Make sure any surgery is performed in an accredited hospital and, if possible, select a hospital that gives staff privileges (i.e., the right to practice in the hospital) to both your doctor and surgeon. The Joint Commission on Accreditation of Hospitals (J.C.A.H.) certifies that institutions it accredits meet certain minimum requirements designed to assure quality patient care. The standards of the J.C.A.H. are not notably high, but they do disqualify the least-adequate hospitals and the out-and-out "butcher shops."

Osteopathic hospitals may be accredited by their own group—the American Osteopathic Association or by the J.C.A.H.

About a fourth of the nation's hospitals are not accredited by the J.C.A.H. or the American Osteopathic Association, but almost all of the better hospitals are. There are about 1,600 unaccredited institutions out of a total of about 7,000 short-term hospitals.

The address of the Joint Commission on Accreditation of Hospitals is 645 North Michigan Avenue, Chicago, Illinois 60611. The address of the American Osteopathic Association is 212 East Ohio Street, Chicago, Illinois 60611.

Another method of assuring quality hospital and surgical care is to make sure the hospital you go to is affiliated with a medical school, and your doctor and surgeon are on the staff of that hospital. Medical school hospitals and their affiliates have a reputation for excellence, and for keeping their medical staffs on the ball.

### Rule 6

Don't push a doctor to perform surgery on you. If you insist on surgery, even if it is unnecessary, you are likely to find a surgeon willing to perform it.

There are "overtreaters" who are willing to perform unnecessary surgery, so don't ask for trouble.

As Howard R. and Martha E. Lewis note in their book, *The Medical Offenders*:

> *The patients whom overtreaters sell most successfully are neurotic women. A gynecologist new to this country observed: "In Europe it is all the doctor can do to persuade a woman to have a needed operation. In America it is difficult to dissuade her from having an unnecessary one."*
>
> *Some women have had six, nine, or 16 major operations in search of relief from their anxiety, malaise, and all-around misery of emotional immaturity.*

One doctor has suggested that females are subjected to unnecessary surgery more often than males because of the male dominance of the

medical profession. Dr. Francis S. Norris, a surgical pathologist, tiates this point of view by citing a 1969 Surgeons' Cancer Conf which it was agreed that surgeons think twice about orchidector cal removal of a testicle), but rarely hesitate to remove an ov

Occasionally a surgeon is overheard to say: "Surgery was u but if I didn't do it, someone else would. And at least I did a Don't be so eager for surgery that you prescribe your own operation.

### Rule 7

Make sure your doctor and surgeon explain both the surgery and the possible benefits and complications of su

Any doctor or surgeon should do so, and you'll be able intelligent decision on surgery when you have the facts. fact, a doctor who fails to disclose the risks of surgery m up to a malpractice suit. Under the legal doctrine of inf patient who has not been fairly advised about the risks legally consented to it. He may, therefore, sue any doc who operates on him without fairly disclosing the risl

All kinds of possible complications may arise from s Dr. Robert E. Rothenberg, in his book *Understandir* complications:

(1)  Pneumonia, once feared, now largely contro

(2)  Embolism (blood clot).

(3)  Postoperative shock.

(4)  Wound infections.

(5)  Postoperative hemorrhage and wound rup

Another serious complication that should be rest.

The risks of surgery depend on many factors dition, and the nature of the operation to be always there, and you're entitled to know prec all the advances in surgery, one out of every surgery alive, according to Dr. Rothenberg. the expected mortality for any given opera higher.

It is true that some minor procedures negligible risk. The uncomplicated remov

in the hands of a surgeon or doctor who engages in such unethical activity. So, politely question any excessive fees to the surgeon's assistant if fee-splitting is suggested. According to the Lewis' book, *The Medical Offenders*, fee-splitting is especially widespread in Pennsylvania.

## Rule 9

Check the surgeon out with those who know him or have used him. This includes other patients as well as associates of the surgeon.

You might want to check on his background in the Directory of Medical Specialists. What school did he go to? Where did he take his residency? How long has he practiced, etc.?

One good way to find the best surgeon is to find out who doctors use when they need surgery for themselves or their families. The greatest compliment to a surgeon is when he is used by a doctor or his family.

Check the surgeon out yourself. You've got to have confidence in him. You don't have to like him, but you should have confidence in him—or find another surgeon.

## Rule 10

Make sure the surgeon knows and is willing to work with your general practitioner or internist. To assure complete, continuous and quality care, close cooperation between the surgeon and your doctor is vital.

If they can't work as a team, you may be the loser.

## Rule 11

Consider a surgeon who is part of a group practice, and preferably a group that includes internists, surgeons and other specialists. This involves doctors who work together on all their cases, and freely consult and communicate with each other.

With a group practice, you are more likely to have a doctor available at all times who is familiar with your case and you have the built-in benefits of consultation.

Some patients are critical of group practice, however, if they get a feeling that they are being passed from one doctor to another.

Group practice takes many forms. It includes partnerships of many kinds, private clinics, and groups sponsored by labor and management.

One type of group practice is the Health Maintenance Organization (HMO). In most HMO's, the surgeon's income does *not* depend on the number of operations he performs. Under the HMO concept, doctors, including surgeons, are paid as much for keeping you well as they are for treating you when you are sick.

A good HMO performs about 50 percent less surgery on its patients than a health insurance plan which compensates doctors on a per case basis. As a result, membership in a good HMO may help save you from unnecessary surgery.

## Rule 12

Select a surgeon who is not too busy to give patients enough time and attention. Surgeons who handle too many cases are bad news for the patient for obvious reasons.

The best surgeons are likely to be busy. But the "best" surgeon who must rush through an operation and must hurry past his patients is not likely to get good results. To say haste makes waste is a gross understatement when discussing surgery.

It may be difficult for you to decide if a surgeon is too busy. You can get some feel for this by observing how crowded his waiting room is and how much time he is willing to spend with you.

## Rule 13

Be especially on guard if some of the operations that are most often unnecessarily performed are proposed for you. These include hysterectomies, hemorrhoidectomies and tonsillectomies. These operations have been referred to as "remunerectomies" by some cynics (a fancy Greek derivative from the word "remuneration"). One doctor, Norman S. Miller of the University of Michigan, coined the term "hip-pocket hysterectomies" because the "only benefactor is the surgeon's wallet." (Philadelphia *Evening Bulletin*, June 8, 1972, page 25.)

## Rule 14

The patient, not the doctor or surgeon, is supposed to, and is entitled to make the decision on whether to have surgery. Listen to the experts. But remember, it's still your decision. You're entitled to have the facts you need, and you're entitled to decide whether or not to go ahead with the surgery.

As the title of the television show goes—"This Is Your Life."

# Index

Abandonment, 241; by husband, 222–24; by wife, 224–27
Abortion, 152, 153, 202; D and C, 199; natural/spontaneous, 150
Abstinence, 157
Achievement: aspiration gap, 28, 29; cultural expectations, 27–28, 29
Actresses, 42, 45, 75, 247, 255–56
Adolescence, 1, 3, 159
*Adrenogenital syndrome,* 15
Adultery, 219, 227–29
Adult-oriented systems, 63
Advertising (ads), 29–30, 49, 64, 243; appealing to women, 243–44; cosmetic, 52; drug, 133, 143, 144; estrogen, 126, 130, 190; laxatives, 125; for singles, 218; valium, 164
Aegean Sea, 143
Aetilus, 104
Affairs, extramarital, 19, 56, 59, 117, 228
Affinal relatives, 218
Affluent societies, 182; nonproductive poor, 256
Africa, 40, 73, 85, 101, 159; dress, 43; Eastern, 13; independence movements, 255; modern society, 254–55; North, 61; Rift Valley, 143; South, 8, 105; West, 18, 41, 101–2, 254–55; women, 254
Afterlife, 89, 172
Age, 2, 21; bias in hiring, 110; Confucian doctrine of respect, 83; double standard, 163 ff.; dress symbols, 43; illnesses, 179; mood, relationship, 256
Aged, the, *vii*, 2, 8, 55, 59; broken hips, 190; emotional needs, 90; problem, 90; status, 40, 57, 60, 62–63, 251
Age group, moving to another status, 54, 57
Aging, 22–23; cultural, 153; delaying,

129, 170; physiology of, 175; preparation for, 252; process, 105, 249–58; standards-values, 49; trauma, 172
Airline stewardesses, 109–10
Air pollution, 183, 193
Air travel, 110, 254
Alberta, 193
Alcohol (alcoholism), 37, 160, 189; abuse, 142
Algeria, 74
Alikeshiev, P. A., 23
Alimony, 217, 222, 231, 241, 242–43, 244
Aloneness (being alone), 217–48; adultery, 227–29; being left, 222–24; divorce: getting, 229–33, and sex, 236–37; loneliness, 233–36; making it alone, 240–48; preparation for, 241; widowhood and sex, 236–37; women who leave, 224–27
Altitude: -menopause/menstruation relationship, 109–10
Alvarez, Dr. Walter, 203
Amenorrhea, 116
American Cancer Society, 187, 196
American College of Obstetricians and Gynecologists, 193–94, 201
American College of Physicians, 214
American College of Surgeons, 214
American dream, 27–30
American Hospital Association, 214
*American Journal of Psychiatry,* 161
American Medical Association (AMA), 214; *Archives of Surgery,* 209, 272, 273; ethical rules, 210; Principles of Medical Ethics, 275; publications, 272, 273
American Osteopathic Association, 215, 276
American Osteopathic Board of Surgery, 273
American society: characteristics, 27,

47; hot springs, 189; marriage, 222; role-playing, 171
Greed, 201
Grief, 36–37, 245, 246
Grooming, 44 ff.; function, 48; industry, 43; marriage, 91; sex, 48; social stimulants, 49
Group practice (physicians), 213
Growing older, 249–58. *See* Aging
Guatemala Indians, 42
Guilt, 86, 90, 95, 168, 256; death, 245
Guttmacher, Dr. Alan, 195
Gynecologists, 11, 15, 111, 128, 145, 158, 162, 166–67, 170, 187, 201, 203, 209
Gynecology: textbooks, 14, 138, 192; operations, 208; problems, 181
Gypsies, 41–42, 124; childbearing, 149–50

Hair (care), 40, 43, 50, 51; danger, 52
Hamilton Anxiety Scale, 163
Happiness: -mood, as indication, 256; money, 255–56; youth, 256
Harem, 17, 18
*Harper's Bazaar,* 11, 42
Harvard University, 269; Medical School, 138; Sociology Department, 138
Hawley, Dr. Paul R., 269, 273
Headache, 126, 139; migraine, 134, 167, 203
Health, 41, 42–43, 106, 107, 108; community, 269; conversational topic, 143; cosmetics, 52; fashion, 188; men/women, 179; middle age, 177–92: atrophic vaginitis, 187, breast cancer, 183–87, heart attacks, 181–83, osteoporosis, 190–92, urinary and vaginal complaints, 188–90
Health delivery system, 270; cost, 271
Health Maintenance Organization (HMO), 213, 279–80
Hearing problems, 179
Heart conditions, 23, 26, 155, 181–83, 190; cardiac arrest, 277; estrogens, 134; men, 23, 179; open-heart surgery, 26; the Pill, 156–57; precautions, 183; research, 181; sex

difference, 181–82; transplants, 272
Hebrews (ancient), 99, 227, 247; divorce, 223, 244; marriage, 220
Hedonism, 224, 238
Heller, Joseph, 33
Hemorrhage, 194, 199, 277
Hemorrhoidectomies, 280
Hepatitis, 194
Heredity, 183
High blood pressure, 179
Hildegard of Bingen, 104–5
Hindus (India), 226–27
"Hip pocket" hysterectomy, 208, 280
Hippocratic Oath, 145
Hite Report, 236
Hoffman-LaRoche, 164
Homeostasis, 123, 124
Homosexuals (homosexuality), 33–36
"Honeymoon cystitis," 189
Hoover, Dr. Robert N., 184
Hopi Indians, 27, 84; divorce, 231–32
Hormones, 109, 119, 126, 129, 161, 165, 191; advertising, *vii;* assays, 104; balance, 118, 120, 122, 127, 128, 198, the Pill, 157; changes, 174; FSH, 119; imbalance, 122–23, 194; male, 36; production, 197; psychology interplay, 23; sex, 23, 183; therapy, 134, 184, 191. *See* Estrogens
Horney, Karen, 168
Hospitals, 214, 243; accreditation, 214–15, 275–76; medical school, 276; mental, 160; number in U.S., 215; osteopathic, 215, 276
Hot flushes, 56, 115, 120, 123–26, 129, 134, 136, 137, 139, 144; cultural component, 124–25; estrogen, 144; psychosomatic component, 124; treatment, 125–26, 138, 185
Housewife: dress, 48–49; role, 69, 93–99, 257; London study, 93–94, 98
"Housewives' disease," 95
Housing, 241, 242, 246–47, 256; study, 255
*Human Sexual Inadequacy,* 14
Human Sexuality Center, 11–12
*Human Sexual Response,* 13